Reshape Your Health

✦

A Beginner's Guide to Getting Fit with No Money, Muscles, or Motivation

✦

Christine Oakes

The information in this book is meant to supplement, not replace, proper exercise training. All forms of exercise pose some inherent risks. The writer, publisher, and editors advise readers to take full responsibility for their safety and know their limits. Before practicing the exercises in this book, be sure that your equipment and exercise environment are safe for use. Do not take risks beyond your level of experience, aptitude, training, and fitness. The exercise and dietary programs in this book are not intended as a substitute for any exercise routine or dietary program that may have been prescribed by your doctor. As with all exercise and dietary programs, you should get your doctor's approval prior to beginning.

Mention of specific companies, organizations, public figures, or authorities in this book does not imply endorsement by the author or publisher, nor does mention of specific companies, organizations, public figures, or authorities imply that they endorse this book, its author, or the publisher.

Internet addresses and company product information given in this book were accurate at the time of publication.

Book design by Eric Coates
Cover design by Margarita Dimova
Book editor: Sean Sabo

Fun2BeFit - Silicon Valley
Training. Yoga. Fitlife.
Your healthy life starts here!

For more information about services and products go to: www.fun2befit.org

Dedication

There are a multitude of people that have helped shape my life and lead me down this road of health and wellness. I know it will be impossible for me to remember everyone, but know that your love, guidance, and encouragement from all of you have not gone unnoticed. I would be a total jerk if I did not first thank my parents Sidney and Connie Oakes. You have both believed in me from the very moment that I popped into this world. Any time I wanted to try something new you said yes. When I failed, you would ask me if it was something important to me. If it was you would tell me to keep trying. You let me stay out until it was dark so I could run outside with the neighborhood kids playing kickball, dodgeball, ride my bike, climb trees, and just be a wild child in the breeze. Thank you for showing me that life only has the limitations that you set upon yourself. If you have heart, desire, and gratitude that you can find happiness anywhere you look because we are all surrounded by it. You just need to open your eyes and see.

To all of my fitness instructors out there, we are changing and inspiring others to lead healthier and longer lives. Thank you for inspiring me to take care of myself when I am too tired to do so. Sharing your creativity influences me in many ways so I can go on to help others when I feel burned out. As a community, we depend on each other to build each other up so we can continue to make a positive impact in this world. Specifically, my mentors Herman Chan, Beverly Hosford, Linda McGrath, Cindy Walker, and Amber Henzi. Thank you for always believing in me more than I believed in myself and seeing that we all have something to contribute in our own unique light.

Lastly, hugs and kisses go out to all of those friends, clients and significant others that supported and believed in me as a fitness professional. From long work days and weeks to referring others to reach out to me to receive my expert advice or services. Your trust in me goes a very long way and I promise that I always have your well-being held close to my heart. As a community, I love how you take what I teach you and share it with others dear to you. Nothing more warms my soul.

~CEO~

Table of Contents

Introduction

Let's cut to the chase. It's pretty obvious why you picked up this book. It isn't because there is some fancy celebrity on the cover who has an airbrushed bod you are gawking over. Or because of a promise that if you only eat meat and veggies or drink lemon juice and cayenne pepper that the pounds will drop off. No, what drove your fingers to open this book is because you know you want to get healthy and aren't sure where to start, but you don't want to do some ridiculous diet or advanced workout plan. The good news is I got you covered!

As a longtime personal trainer and yoga instructor, I have worked with so many different types of people. It is actually one of the things that I love about my job. Many of my clients are busy business professionals such as doctors, lawyers, writers, and engineers. On the flip side, I also have a handful of clients that are stay-at-home moms or dads who also have very limited time between soccer practices and dance recitals. Then there is the client that fits into both of these categories. Bravo to those that have a demanding career and raise a family. These clients have such big hearts to put so much time and energy into two things that they are very passionate about. ALL of these clients came to me because they didn't know how or where to start. Sound like you?

I'm here to tell you that it is completely possible to get healthy. I have seen many of my clients go on to achieve their fitness goals with my workouts as well as the nutritional guidance that I give them. The idea is to start simple. You will find that if you just make small changes, that it not only seems possible, but it is actually easy. This guide is not about achieving a six-pack. Personally, I have no desire ever to have one. Having a ripped body is all about extreme dieting, extreme workouts, and extreme misery. This book is a way to get you fit enough to achieve your first 5K race, help reduce belly bloat, and give you more energy so you can chase after your kids or grandkids.

There are only 3 things that you need to get started:
1. The desire to get healthier
2. An understanding that you may have setbacks
3. Knowing that there is a fit and healthy person inside of you waiting to burst out

What you are going to find in this book is a step-by-step guide on ways you can start to exchange time to make room for healthier food, get more exercise, and improve the quality of your life. You will not find any extreme diets, Olympic lifts, or empty promises. I believe in being realistic in setting fitness goals (we will talk later on how to set reasonable goals) so that you feel successful about what you are doing and begin living a healthy lifestyle. In my experience, people tend to give up when they feel that all of their efforts are not working because the bar they have set for themselves is totally out of reach. Don't let this be you. Continue on to discover the fun ways you can create a fit life for yourself.

Part 1:

The Mindset

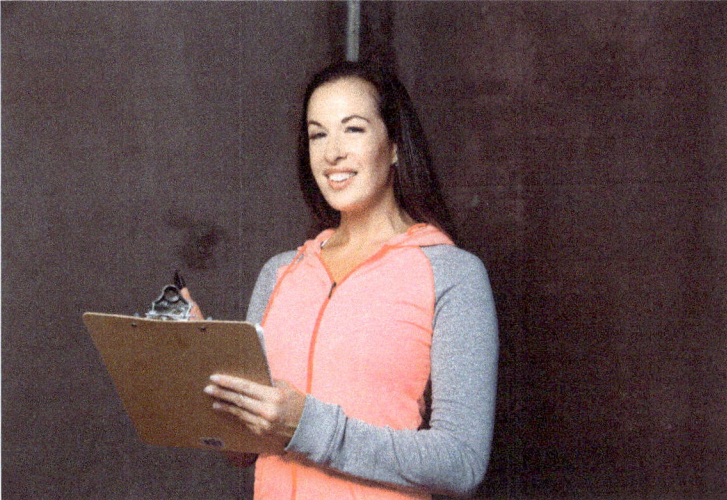

Let's Get Started!

Healthy or Ripped?

Does one represent the other? Are people in the gym or on magazine covers who are completely shredded healthy? I'm here to tell you that they may be and they may not be. For some, the goal is to have a six-pack or completely flat stomach that they can prance around on the beach with. However, it is also possible to achieve this ripped look in an extremely unhealthy way.

As an ACE-certified Health Coach, I can tell you that a healthy body fat range for women is 25 to 31% and for men, it is 18 to 24%. Just to give you an example of how a six-pack look reflects upon someone's health, the amount of essential fat needed for women is 10 to 13%. This range is the level necessary for a woman's body to function properly.

Women who compete in figure competitions perform with typically around a 6 to 10% body fat range. Such a range is achieved by maintaining an athletic body composition and then taking extreme measures of water restriction and crash dieting prior to competition to shed even more fat. If you ask me, this sounds absolutely horrible. Being in the fitness industry, I have spoken to those people that have done this, and they say how utterly miserable they were. They had major headaches, increased irritability, and they seriously hated every moment. Sadly enough, we as a society think that this look is standard for someone that is fit. Total bull!!!! It is so far from the truth.

What Does It Mean to Be Fit?

Being fit has so many different definitions depending on who you talk to. To me, being fit is working out three to five times per week, eating mostly plant-based food, and being able to functionally move my body with push-ups, squats, lunges, and pull-ups. For many, how you define being fit depends on your current state of physical fitness. If you aren't currently participating in a wellness program, you may find that eating more veggies and going for a walk a few times a week will make you feel fitter. On the other hand, if you eat fairly clean (which we will discuss later does not involve washing your food) and do cardio a few times a week, then you may be looking to up your game a bit.

~~~~~*Defining* YOUR *Fit*~~~~~

Start a journal to write down what it would mean to you for you to feel fit. Understand that this can change over time as you begin to live a healthier lifestyle. Consider where you would like to be one year from now. Write down today's date, your name, "Fun2BeFit Life", and the current year/next year (unless you are starting on January 1st). Take those ideas that have been bouncing around in your head about what that you would look like and list them. Don't go all crazy with it. Just a few things will do.

Here's my list for the upcoming year:
1. Eat a plant-based diet with 2 to 3 servings of fruits and veggies per meal every day.
2. Use Yoga Tune-Up balls 2 or more times per week to alleviate shoulder tension.
3. Take my exercise outdoors 2 to 3 times a month to promote excitement into my workouts.
4. Work on handstands in weekly yoga classes to confidently hold unassisted in 6 months.
5. Only take on as much work as is realistic on a daily basis so I can achieve 7 to 8 hours of average sleep within 6 months to a year.

Now it's your turn. Give yourself some time and know that these items can change at any given moment. As a matter of fact, you may just switch things up a bit as you continue reading through this book. Feel free to record your goals here or in a private journal.

Fun2BeFit Goals for 20___/20___.

1. _____

2. _____

3. _____

4. _____

5. _____

As you will see from my goals, there are not any workout goals. I have established pretty consistent habits of working out; therefore, my focus has shifted to other things that I know would make me happier and healthier. You will find that from year to year your own definition of what fit is and how you want to get there will constantly evolve. Once specific goals become a regular part of your life, you will graduate and focus on new things.

~~~~~~

Are Your Goals SMART?

We aren't looking for thick glasses and a pocket protector here. There are certain characteristics that will differentiate your goals from being successful ones to something that may set you up for failure. While some goals you may set for yourself may not happen as planned (that's why I have you make 5), you can create goals that are within arm's reach as long as you are consistent with your approach.

Review your goals and modify them to make sure they fit within the SMART criteria:

S - Check that your goals are *specific*. If you want to lose weight, then how much do you want to lose? What size do you want to be?
M - Can you *measure*, in some way, what you want to achieve? Frequency? Pounds? Inches? Time? It's important to be able to track your progress so you can feel the success.
A - Please make sure that the goals you seek out are *attainable*. It's great to be ambitious, but sometimes it is helpful to take a lofty goal and create mini-goals. You will have more times to celebrate success along the way.
R - This one seems obvious, but you want to focus on things that are *realistic* to your desires, abilities, and needs. If you aspire to run a marathon, it would be logical to start off with training for a 5K.

T - If you never had a deadline for something or could just show up for an appointment whenever you felt like it, would anything ever get accomplished? Probably not. If you create *time*-bound objectives for yourself, it will be easier to review and tweak things along the way so you can see what works and what doesn't.

Sometimes, life changes like getting married, having a job change, or having kids, and these things can have you reverting back to old goals. That's ok! Life happens and will get in the way. If you find yourself slipping, just reassess your goals and hop back onto the saddle. It's not the end of the world. You were strong enough to achieve your goals once, and you sure as hell can do it again. I believe in you. Now, you just have to believe in yourself.

~~~~~*Investing In Your Health*~~~~~

Kalenga "Kay" Pembamoto is a single 29-year-old living in California currently exploring different career paths. Kay and I know each other from my donation-based yoga-in-the-park classes that she found on the website MeetUp.com. She mentioned that for her, "To be fit is to invest in the long-term quality of my life. Whether it's going for an extra walk during a particularly slow-moving day or passing up binge drinking to curl up with some hot tea, I value taking small steps that make me feel good inside and out." At a pivotal point in her career of finding something that is going to give her long-term financial security, Kay looks at her health with that same focus. To her, staying fit means that she is funding her health bank to use in her later years just as much as her 401k will do the same for her financially.

~~~~~

Sprinkles

Sorry, but these are not the cupcake-kind. Don't scrunch your face in disappointment! Since each of you are all starting off fitness at different levels with your own set of challenges, you will want to find ways that you can add in "sprinkles" here and there to get you closer to where you want to be. If you attempt to do a complete overhaul of your health right off the bat, there is a really good chance that it will be too overwhelming and you will quit before you even get started. Yoga instructors use this term a lot when teaching classes. You take a theme or concept, and then just add in bits and pieces throughout the class. It doesn't consume the entire hour, but you have these little reminders here and there that connect the dots to pull everything together.

I coach my clients to just sprinkle healthy things in throughout their day. Maybe if you go out for lunch, you opt for the side salad instead of fries. If you have a meeting with your boss, see if they would be up for doing a walking meeting and getting in some fresh air. Sprinkles represent these tiny ways that you can inch closer to the healthy person you want to ultimately become. How can you sprinkle in healthy changes into your day? You can even plan your sprinkles ahead of time while showering or brushing your teeth in the morning!

Why Are You Doing This?

This question is an important one to ask and understand. If you are doing this out of societal pressure to look a certain way, just stop. That is a completely asinine way of thinking. Most of everything that is in the media these days is fake. Seriously! It really makes me sick that people are "fixed" to appear more desirable. Someone that is a total inspiration to me and has fueled my drive to want to succeed in the fitness industry is Jillian Michaels. You may know her from *The Biggest Loser*, which is where I first became drawn to her as an inspirational role model. She also records a weekly podcast, *The Jillian Michaels Show*, which I enjoy from time to time.

One day as I was listening to her podcast, Michaels openly admitted that she has cellulite on the back of her thighs, just like me. Someone that I admire completely who is in the media and looks fantastic in any photo that I've ever seen ... is an actual human with flaws. Hearing her say this was such a relief to me at the time because I was new to the fitness industry and was really worried about looking the part of a trainer. Her being able to admit that even she had flaws made me realize that each of us will never be perfect. Or maybe we already are in our own way.

When I stopped trying to focus on looking a certain way and honed in on what was important, that is when I truly started to feel comfortable and happy with who I was. Instead of trying to mold myself into something I wasn't, I started thinking about what my real motivation was for wanting to be healthy. It is so, so very important that you consider why you are doing this.

- •. Do you have family that you want to be more involved with? Do you want to run with your kids?
- •. Do you physically want to be able to take care of an elderly parent?
- •. Do you want to be able to go out with your friends for a hike or walk around town without feeling exhausted?
- •. Do you want more energy to put time into growing your career?
- •. Are you on a ton of medication and want to live a drug-free life?

We all have things that are important to us, and it differs from one person to the next. For me, I would like to live a long and pain-free life. Both sides of my family have a history of cancer, high blood pressure, and high cholesterol. The start of my journey began with me quitting smoking after 11 years of puffing on those cancer sticks. It was just not in line with my goals, and I surely did not want to suffer or die at a very young age like my smoker grandparents. As a lover of international travel, I hope that I will have many years to discover ancient history, explore different cuisines, and connect with many interesting people all across the globe.

It's time to get real with yourself. Allow yourself to be vulnerable and honest. The sooner you can do that, the quicker you will be on your way to becoming a healthier version of who you are today.

Your Why Matters

Take a moment to think about why you picked up this book. Having these constant reminders will be a great reference when you are having a hard time getting motivated or staying on track.

- •. Why do you want to become healthier?
- •. What and who is important to you?
- •. How do you want to feel about yourself?

~~~~~Create Your Board of Reason~~~~~

You just identified why you are doing this. Now it is time to create a board that will be a constant reminder. It's similar to a vision board but a bit different. To me, a vision board is something that you dream of having. Your "Board of Reason" is compiled of things that are important to you now and that you want to keep in your life. It is your motivation when you need to be reminded why you want to make changes in your life. You will look at this board and tell yourself to get it together. These people and these things on your Board of Reason are just something you never want to lose because of unhealthy choices in your life. You don't need to have a huge science project-type board. Just have something that is enough to serve as a constant reminder as well as support.

Things you will want to fill in your Board of Reason are things you already possess:

- •. Family
- •. Friends
- •. Maybe a race bib from previous race
- •. A photo of you being happy
- •. Your favorite vacation spot
- •. An accomplishment you are proud of
- •. Anything else that is important to you

~~~~~~

My Top 5 Things You Can Do Today to Be a Healthier Version of You

1.Veggies

Eat them at 2 to 3 of your meals daily. Start by sticking with the ones that you love. For me, that is spinach, mushrooms, tomatoes, corn, asparagus, Brussels sprouts, broccoli, eggplant, and zucchini. I was a very weird child, so if you only like 1 or 2 to start, that is fine. Veggies are loaded with tons of nutrients and can have a powerful impact on your inner health. The more variety of colors, the more variety of nutrients you end up consuming. Think of a rainbow when you are eating throughout the week. It doesn't have to be all in 1 meal or 1 day. Just place them here and there in your meals as your week progresses.

2. **Water**
Carry it with you all day, every day. I am a horrible water drinker, but if I have it with me, I will constantly sip on it. Daily, you want to consume about half of your body weight in ounces of water. For example, I weigh 130 pounds, so I would want to shoot for a minimum of 65 ounces of water per day. Remember to drink more water when you workout. Generally speaking, an additional 12 to 16 ounces of water will be enough for every hour of a workout. I like to sip throughout my entire workout for better absorption and to avoid that sloshing feeling in your stomach as you exercise.

3. **Move**
There will be times that you will only have 20 minutes to do something. I always tell my clients that something is better than nothing. If you don't have as much time, then try to push yourself a little more than you typically would. Remind yourself how good your body feels when you go for a walk, get on a bike, or do strength training.

4. **Sleep**
Sleep can actually be one of the more challenging things for most people. Kids or no kids, we tend to be in a go, go, go society. Throw in tablets, cell phones, and streaming your favorite shows that all give your brain added stimulation instead of relaxation before bed. I will provide you with tips later on how to improve your quality of sleep and how it can directly correlate to maintaining a healthy weight.

5. Meditation

If you can meditate once a week to start, it will be enough to start noticing the benefits. Personally, I like to do guided meditation either at the end of a yoga class or with a meditation app on my phone. The two apps that I recommend are "Calm" and "Headspace" (more info in the reference list section at the back of the book). Both are FREE with upgrade options but will be good enough to get you started. The meditations are short and give you the opportunity to put your brain on pause. As stated above, we have constant stimulation coming at us all day long. Recharge your day and step away for just a few moments. I promise you that whatever is pressing will still be there when you are finished in 5 minutes. You just may be able to address whatever it is with more focus and attention.

~~~~~ Take Control ~~~~~

Julia, a 35-year-old engineer from Ludlow, Massachusetts, is truly someone with drive and motivation. She was diagnosed with fibromyalgia around 2 years ago. As a means to control her discomfort, her doctor prescribed exercise for her. When speaking with Julia, she told me that when she was initially diagnosed she "was miserable both physically and mentally. My doctor recommended exercise as one way to help with the pain, but that felt impossible. I decided to try yoga, and over time, I realized that even if I was in pain, I could still take a class. Not only that, but I felt better within a few minutes, and sometimes I would feel better for the remainder of the day.

Realizing that aches and pains were not a good excuse for missing a workout, I slowly increased the number of times I would sweat each week. Now 2 years after that diagnosis, I am stronger than I have ever been. My pain from fibromyalgia has decreased considerably. I am more likely to be sore from a good workout than from my illness. Not all days are easy, but I know it is important to keep the momentum going if I want to keep feeling good."

Julia is truly an inspirational story. I first met her in my yoga classes and then she got brave enough to join my boot camp classes. She does not slack at all and puts her best effort in when attending class. It is quite evident that Julia not only believes in the process but also believes in her health and well-being.

~~~~~~

Visualizing a Healthy You

Part of turning into this more fit version of yourself is being able to imagine yourself doing things that may seem impossible or far out of reach. Close your eyes and imagine yourself as this amazing avatar that embodies all of the things you want to do physically. Your avatar is going for hikes, throwing the kids around, and eating more fruits and veggies. It can be anything you want it to be.

~~~~~Journal Time~~~~~

Remember a time in your life that you felt healthy, fit, or active.
- •. How old were you?
- •. What did it feel like in your body?
- •. Was it easy or challenging to maintain?
- •. What are ways that you can sprinkle in changes to get closer to returning to this healthier you?

Now go out and be this person! Not tomorrow. Not next week. Start today! You totally got this, and know that I've got your back.

~~~~~

Things to Remember

- •. Remember that being fit to you doesn't necessarily look like what it does in magazines or social media. Fit is not defined by physical aesthetics.
- •. Remind yourself what you are working towards. Know your purpose.
- •. Reflect on your Board of Reason. The people, things, and ambitions that you have are important. No matter how big or small they may seem.
- •. Sprinkles everywhere! It sounds fun like you are tossing confetti around but just in the form of a healthy lifestyle. These are small little pieces that will eventually make an overall larger impact on your health.
- •. Be able to see yourself as this new healthy person. Don't be afraid to take on this newfound person with confidence. Be ready to have others try to sway you away and refer back to the above to explain to those close to you why this is so important and ask for their support.

Part 2:
What We Eat

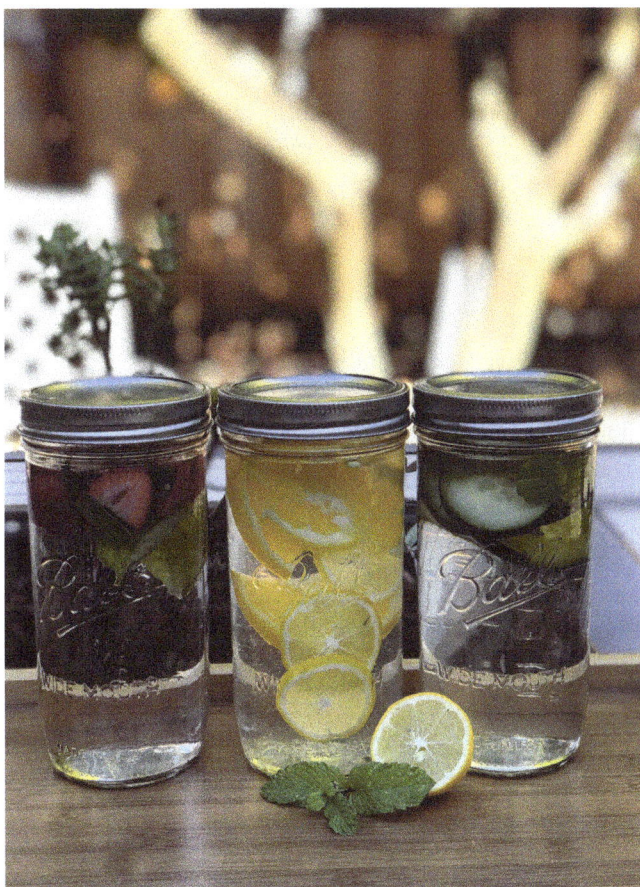

Friend or Foe

One of the trickiest things for most people to maneuver is the topic of food. We are constantly bombarded by things in the media about eating more of this and avoiding that because it causes cancer. Eat more veggies right? Well, no kidding! When I first became a professional in the industry, I too was confused by all of the contradictory information that was out there. What do I tell my clients to eat or not eat to guide them in the right direction?

The fact of the matter is that although many personal trainers give out specific nutrition advice, meal plans, and tell their clients to avoid or consume certain foods, it is completely out of my scope of practice as a personal trainer. What I can do is share with you my findings through research and my own experiences so you can experiment with what works best for you. After all, diet and exercise is not a one-size-fits-all approach.

No Six-Pack Here ... I Like To Cheat!

So here's the thing: I get it. I'm a trainer, and I am supposed to have this amazing body, have an unlimited amount of self-control, and to snub at anyone that decides to have dessert. The truth is that I am a human being just like you. Of course, I want dessert and cheese and all of the other things that are not suppose to be good for you. Except for mayo ... that stuff just grosses me out. Ick!!!

Where I have seen it go wrong for my clients is that they have a cheat day instead of a cheat meal. If you had a slice of pizza once a week, you are not going to turn into a morbidly obese person as long as the rest of your week is balanced out with veggies, lean protein, healthy fats, and complex carbs.

Flip the script, and let's say you go out for a fantastic brunch with eggs Benedict, hash browns, and 2 mimosas. Screw it! Have 3 mimosas cause it's your cheat day, right?!?!?! Lunch rolls around, and it's time for Mexican. We have guacamole and chips to start. Then we have some enchiladas smothered in gooey cheese, but we'll do veggies so we don't feel too guilty. The margaritas at this place are boooomb! Of course you're having a second so you can have more time with your friends. After all of that day-drinking, you are too tired to cook, so you just go home and eat a Caesar salad for dinner. The salad makes up for the rest of the cheat day, right?

Here's the math:
    Breakfast - 1,343 kcal
    Lunch - 1.499 kcal
    Dinner - 360 kcal
    Grand total of ... drum roll, please ... 3,202 kcal

Unless you are an extreme athlete, this caloric intake is likely to wipe out all of your efforts from the week. Not to mention the lack of nutrients. Why do that to yourself? It would suck to work so hard to eat well and sweat bullets in the gym all week to just ruin everything in one day right? Look, I'm not saying you can never have these foods; you just need to go easy. If you really want the mimosas, then go with a veggie egg scramble and a side of fruit. Want the enchiladas? Skip the margaritas or have a shot of tequila on the rocks and skip the sugar. It's all about shifting things around so you still feel like you can enjoy your time out and can socialize without feeling socially awkward or like you are depriving yourself.

The Other 23 Hours

So you get a workout buddy or personal trainer, and you totally kill it in your workout. Typically, it's not about all of your good doings during that solid workout sesh, but the time you spend when you step away and go on with your day-to-day responsibilities. You have a deadline on a project, you need to take the kids from here to there, you have to pay the bills, do the laundry, and the list goes on.

Stress can wreak havoc on your diet, and the best thing you can do is be prepared. Remember, it is not always about having this perfect plan and making amazing meals every day. If you can figure a way to sprinkle in a bit of nutrient-dense foods here and there, then you will be moving in a path towards a healthier lifestyle. As you eat, start to think if you can add something to your meal or remove something that will make it healthier. How about adding chopped veggies to your eggs? Or add avocado instead of cheese to your salad? How about switching in whole wheat or quinoa pasta instead of white pasta?

Here Are My Top 5 Food Hacks to Avoid the Fast Food Wagon:

1. **Have healthy snacks on hand**: Many days, I am training clients from 7 in the morning until 10 at night. It is not uncommon for me to have to go long periods between meals, but I would be the world's biggest biotch of a trainer if I didn't carry snacks with me. I always have something along the lines of a Kind bar, trail mix, or veggies and hummus. The first 2 are the easiest since they don't need re-frigeration. For things that need to stay cool, I like to use my chilled lunchbox by PackIt. It has built-in cooling packs for no fuss, and they come in all different sizes.

2. **Make meals in bulk**: I don't have kids, but I barely have time to cook due to my demanding schedule. Many of us are pressed for time with a multitude of responsibilities. You can make soups, stews, chilis, and my Mexican quinoa in bulk and then freeze half of it for a later date. Do this on your day off and make it the meal you are cooking for that day. Just double the recipe! My trick to save space in the freezer is to put half of the meal in a freezer storage bag and lay it on a cookie sheet to freeze flat. Once it is frozen, you will have a meal in a bag that is stackable, and you can defrost when you are ready to enjoy.

3. **Purchase pre-chopped fruits and veggies**: Today, we are so lucky to be able to go to the store and buy fresh produce that is prepped and ready to go. You can buy the unprepped fruit or veggie to do it yourself, but if you are short on time, it is not much more to buy it ready-to-go. Whether you are in a food desert or not, you may also find these items available in the freezer section if you want to stock up over the long haul. Frozen fruits are great for smoothies, and frozen veggies are great for stir-frys, soups, and pasta bakes. Stock up on these items to save you time and trim your waistline.

4. **Know where to go in a pinch**: Sometimes all of the preparation in the world will still leave you between a rock and a hard spot. Know your go-tos if you are left with minimal options. For me, if I either ran out of my emergency snacks or am super short on time, I will:
  •. Go to a Thai restaurant and get a veggie curry (whichever has the largest array of veggies) with brown rice.
  •. Get a Chipotle salad with no dressing and extra veggies, black beans, mild salsa (for the chunky tomatoes), and guacamole.
  •. Go to a Subway for a salad with avocado and light vinaigrette dressing.
  •. Go to a grocery store and get a rotisserie chicken, microwaveable frozen veggies, and microwaveable brown rice.Know what you have access to and where you can get it. I find that if you are in dire straits, the less thinking you have to do, the better choices you will make. Have an emergency backup plan that you can easily fall back on.

5. **Keep the junk out**: This is advice that I give to all of my clients. If it is not around you in your home, you are less likely to cave if you have a moment of weakness. Do you really think that you are going to drive to the store at 11 o'clock at night when you are craving ice cream? Not likely. It may sound really good for about 10 minutes, but the moment will pass, and the calories will not be consumed. It is something so simple, yet there are many people that I give this advice to that allow these crappy foods into their homes. It has to be a conscious choice to want to be healthy. If you have others at

home, share with them your why, and they will be onboard to support you too.

Crap Is Whack!

Food addiction is a real thing. Sadly enough, our prominent food corporations are well aware of this and create foods that will keep consumers coming back because they can't get enough. I won't name names, but you can go to the store yourself and identify the companies that make the top-selling potato chips, desserts on the shelf (how come the cream filling doesn't need to be refrigerated?), and easy mac and cheese (again, why doesn't the cheese require refrigeration?).

Look, I'm not going to bullshit you and say I've never had these things, but once I began working in the fitness industry and started researching, I had a true genuine awakening. Just pause for a second and really think about it. How are these "foods" able to last so long in some box on the shelf? The simple answer is that they are NOT real food.

The Fat/Sugar/Salt Triangle

What if I told you that food could have the same effect on you that cocaine or heroin can? Would you think I'm crazy? Or maybe you are thinking how certain foods are difficult to resist. I'm here to tell you that I'm not crazy, and that food addiction is real.

Like I stated previously, there are major food manufacturers that are well aware of the abilities for food with certain properties to hook people into having a constant craving. I'm not kidding. For real, these influential companies use these tactics to fatten their pockets. They state that it is the responsibility of the consumer to know what they are buying and control how much they consume. It's similar to the housing crisis in 2008 when big banks told buyers that their monthly payments were only going to be $1,000 per month, but in the long haul, the payments would be $3,000 per month or more! It's a game of poker; trust only what you can read on the label, and you get bonus points if it is fresh produce with no label. Don't fall into the Bermuda triangle of food. Be knowledgeable about what you eat.

Pantry Reboot:

So you know by now that certain foods are just going to be major roadblocks on where you want to go on your healthy journey. It's time for us to remove those obstacles and create a clearer path for your wellness future.

Step 1: Clear the junk. You know what I'm talking about. All of the obvious crap like cookies, chips, candy, ice cream, and mac and cheese. Just let it go straight into the trash. Keep your canned beans, frozen veggies, pasta sauce, whole grain pasta, vegan soups, peanut butter or almond butter, brown rice, olive oil, avocado oil, coconut oil, and spices.

Step 2: Start reading labels. Notice items that are full of refined sugar, saturated fats, high fructose corn syrup, and high in sodium (it is typically smart to stay away from foods with more sodium than calories per serving), and toss all of these in the trash if you have any in your home. Don't cry, and don't think of donating. Even if you have a tight budget, remind yourself that you are going to start buying budget-friendly healthy foods like frozen veggies. If you know this stuff is terrible for your health, you sure as hell would not want to pass on the disease-laden food to a stranger, would you? That's just all kinds of bad karma, my friend.

Step 3: Stock up on healthy foods you like. You can refer to my shopping list for suggestions on foods that are nutritious. Begin with veggies and fruits that you already know that you enjoy. You can research recipes that include these foods to start off with meals you know you will like.

Do you have picky eaters around? If you have little ones that don't like broccoli or carrots or anything that is good for them, you can set the veggies aside to add to their meals like you would at a taco bar. For example, I like to add a ton of veggies to my pasta so that it is heavier on them. It would be easy enough to just steam or sauté them on the side. When I add pasta to my plate, I can add a large scoop of veggies to the plain pasta. This also gives you the opportunity just to set a tiny bit aside to start introducing these foods to your family. That way you aren't making 2 separate meals which can be a total pain in the booty. Once you start exploring with all kinds of new recipes, you can take your newfound knowledge to sprinkle in the goodness to meals you are accustomed to eating. Plus, I have easy recipes later in the book that will give you ideas to get started. Obviously!

So What Should I Buy?

It is very daunting to think about changing what you eat. Understand that this will not happen overnight, and there will be setbacks. As a gradual lifestyle change, it can be easier to focus on adding in healthier options here and there than to replace the ones that are not good for your body. You are just sprinkling in a bit of healthy here and a little there. Just take it 1 meal at a time and eventually adding in nutrient-dense foods will become second nature.

First, start by focusing on purchasing REAL food. Not those food-like products that are packaged in boxes and last on a shelf for 3 to 5 years. Think apples picked fresh off of a tree or fish straight from the ocean. Or spinach from a field. None of these things have gone through a factory to be manufactured. I have put together things I enjoy eating and created a shopping list for you to reference below. Many of these are things I always have on hand so I am assured that I won't be in a frustrating place without something to eat. Feel free to add in your favorite foods that are similar but that I may not have included on my list.

Things I consider when shopping are the same things I just had you consider as you cleaned out your pantry. Is it high in sodium or saturated fats? Is it nutrient-dense (such as fruits and veggies)? Is it highly processed (most things that are meant to last years on a shelf are and are loaded with preservatives)? This is not to say that you will never have any of these foods again, but you want them to be the exceptions and not the rule. The best way to do so is by keeping the bad foods far away from your house like the plague.

Shopping List

Veggies:
Asparagus
Broccoli
Bok choy
Brussels sprouts
Cabbage
Dark Leafy greens (such as spinach, kale, chard)
Green beans
Mushrooms
Onions
Carrots
Squash
Cucumbers
Bell peppers

Fruits:
Apples
Pears
Strawberries
Raspberries
Oranges
Bananas
Peaches
Mangos

Tomatoes

Avocados

Lemons

Limes

Carbs:

Whole wheat or quinoa pasta

Quinoa

Brown rice

Sweet potatoes

Whole wheat tortillas

Canned Goods:

Pasta sauce (low-sodium)

Diced tomatoes

Beans (such as garbanzo, black, pinto, navy)

Lentils

Soup (low-sodium and preferably dairy-free)

Vegetable/Chicken broth

Peanut or almond butter

Frozen Foods:

Veggies

Fruits

Veggie burgers

Shrimp

Lean ground turkey or beef (preferably grass-fed)

Salmon

Chicken breast

Edamame

Falafel

From the Deli:

Fresh salsa

Hummus

Eggs
Tofu
Dairy-free creamer
Nuts (such as almonds, walnuts, pistachios)
Nut cheese (Miyoko's is my fave)
Chia seed

Seasonings:
Minced garlic
Salt
Pepper
Cilantro
Cayenne
Chili powder
Cinnamon
Cumin

Oils and Condiments:
Avocado oil
Olive oil
Mustard
Balsamic vinegar
Ketchup (without high-fructose corn syrup)
Vinaigrette dressing

~~~~~Journal Time~~~~~

Name 3 meals that you make on a regular basis. What can you add from the shopping list to "sprinkle" a bit of healthy into these meals you already enjoy or remove an ingredient that is not healthy?

1._____

2._____

3._____

Here are some ideas to get you started:
- •. Add veggies into your pasta, such as spinach, mushrooms, asparagus, or squash.
- •. Change out your white pasta for whole wheat or quinoa pasta.
- •. Instead of getting yogurt with fruit (which is loaded with sugar), get plain yogurt and add your own fruit, such as berries.
- •. Swap out your chicken salad sandwich and instead have a grilled chicken sandwich with avocado. This removes all of the unhealthy fat in the mayo and adds good fat from avocado.
- •. For salads, use spinach or a spring mix in lieu of nutrition-less iceberg lettuce. Top with homemade vinaigrette instead of drowning it in a calorie-laden creamy dressing.

Making these small changes will put you in the mindset of healthy without the overwhelming feeling of an overhaul. The goal is not to feel deprived as you would in your standard "diet" and to allow you to see that you are eating just a different version of those satisfying foods.

Organic Doesn't Always Equate to Healthy

Unfortunately, we live in a society where company pockets are deep, and big corporations have a primary focus to maximize sales. Seriously, this sucks for us as consumers because we feel that what is put into the media and backed by the government should be true, right? Luckily, you have taken the first step in the right direction by choosing to educate yourself by reading this book. I am not a registered dietician, but I have done enough research to know that YOU have to be the one to take responsibility for what you eat. Don't rely on the marketing ploys placed on the front of food labels in the store, or it will be a big slap in your face.

With that said, it isn't always necessary to buy organic, especially if you are strapped for cash and you just can't afford it. Isn't it nice to know that you and your family can still be healthy without breaking the bank? Generally, fruits and veggies are fairly inexpensive as long as you shop for foods that are in season. Some produce will likely have a high level of pesticides used on them unless you opt to go the organic route.

The Environmental Working Group keeps an up to date list of produce that is known to have a high level of pesticide usage. You can visit their site at www.ewg.org for the most up-to-date list. For now, here is a list of the "Clean 15 and Dirty Dozen."

Clean 15:
Sweet corn
Avocados
Pineapples
Cabbage
Onions
Sweet peas
Papayas
Asparagus
Mangos
Eggplant
Honeydew melon
Kiwi
Cantaloupe
Cauliflower
Grapefruit

Dirty Dozen:
Strawberries
Spinach
Nectarines
Apples
Peaches
Pears
Cherries
Grapes
Celery
Tomatoes
Sweet bell peppers
Potatoes

Somewhere Over the Rainbow

Judy Garland once sang the song "Over the Rainbow" as Dorothy Gale in *The Wizard of Oz* to reference that the only colorful thing that Dorothy had seen in Kansas was a rainbow. Now that you have cleared out all of the bland-looking foods in your home and filled your pantry with ones full of color, it is time to start creating meals utilizing this vibrancy. Think about it for a second: Have you ever seen a salad, for example, that is made with iceberg lettuce, some cucumber, and a few pieces of tomato? I have, and I can tell you that I will totally snub my nose at it. How boring!! Seriously, don't even feed me that garbage.

Sticking with the salad example, say you have a salad of either spinach or spring greens with quinoa, carrots, strawberries, and avocado. Or maybe cherry and golden tomatoes, cucumber, avocado, and cilantro drizzled with balsamic vinegar? Not all salads need to have lettuce, you know. The point is that the more colors you add to your food, the more appealing it becomes. The more it will tickle your taste buds because of the multitude of flavors you introduce. The bonus is that the more colors you include in your meals throughout the week, the more nutrients you are consuming. The more you "sprinkle" colors into your foods, the more your body will thank you.

Just to give you an idea of the benefits, here is what I call the nutritional rainbow:

Color	Contains	Benefit
Red	lycopene	antioxidant
Orange	beta-carotene	supports immune system; antioxidant

Color	Contains	Benefit
Yellow	vitamin C; flavonoids	detoxifying; inhibits tumor cell growth
Green	folate	builds healthy cells and genetic material
White-green	allyl-sulfides	reduces cell division; supports immune system
Blue	anthocyanins	destroys free radicals
Red-purple	resveratrol	decreases estrogen production
Brown	fiber	removes carcinogens

~~~~~Bros (broccoli) before Carbos (carbohydrates)~~~~~

Uma is an 18-year-old Berkeley undergrad trying to transition from home life to college life. As every college freshman moves away from home, they worry about that dreaded "freshman 15" (students gain 15 pounds on average their first semester in college). Is it preventable or inevitable? When speaking to Uma about staying healthy in college, she stated, "I have become a healthier eater by finding recipes that have lots of vegetables or eating a salad before eating a heavier or carbo-loaded meal. That way, I am more filled up by the vegetables and don't eat as much of the carbohydrates, like rice or pasta.

"I have found that if you eat your veggies first, that is a good way to make sure you get all of the nutrient-dense foods and fill up on less of the other stuff, so you don't overeat. I don't feel deprived since I consume everything in moderation. In the evening, I like to take a shower and sip on a cup of chamomile tea. Making sure I get enough rest ensures that I won't crave junk food before I head to bed."

Uma is an excellent example of how you can still enjoy some of the things that you like, but front-load your meals with the stuff that is good for you to find the appropriate nutritional balance. She isn't focused on removing things from her diet, but she is more focused on eating veggies that she knows that she likes. This way she doesn't feel deprived and yet can eat a primarily nutrient-dense meal.

~~~~~~~

Hitting the Reset Button

Now that you have cleared out your kitchen of the obvious, I have another challenge for you. This is totally up to you ... if you want to take it or leave it, that is your decision. If this is your first attempt to try to get healthy, the kitchen clean-out may be fairly extreme for you, and you will need an adjustment period to get used to having veggies in every meal. That is totally ok. You may or may not come back to this point in the book.

On the other hand, let's say that you knew certain processed foods were not good for you. For the most part, you cook from home, and fast food is not your go-to. Do you have a healthy diet that doesn't need tweaking? Maybe. For the longest time, I thought my food choices were good, and I have had many of clients that say the same about themselves.

The thing is what works for us as individuals can vary from person-to-person. I promised you earlier in the book that I would not have a one-size-fits-all plan. I'm here to tell you that this is so very true. My research over the years has led me to believe that certain foods are inflammatory, acidic, and addictive to our bodies. These foods do not necessarily have the same effect on every individual, but it is worth considering to see if these foods cultivate a negative response based on your body type.

Top Inflammatory, Acidic, and Addictive Foods:

Wheat/Gluten—baked goods, pastas, and cereals
Soy—Meat and dairy alternatives, such as soy milk and tofu
Dairy—Cheese, protein powders, stuffed pastas, etc.
Sugar—Desserts, soda, baked goods, etc.
Alcohol—Beer, wine, and spirits
Coffee-Don't get angry at me just drink green tea ;)

To find out if your body has any adverse effects to these known offenders, I suggest removing these items completely from your diet for at least 1 week. It sounds crazy, I know, but just try it. I removed these types of foods from my meals for a full 30 days and dropped 8 pounds!

My meals were structured as follows:
- •. 50% veggies (any veggies in your fridge)
- •. 25% protein (chicken, fish, turkey, lentils, beans, tempeh)
- •. 25% healthy fats and healthy carbs (avocado, olive oil, and nuts for fats; brown rice, quinoa, and sweet potatoes for carbs)

It doesn't sound like a lot, but mind you I was 5-foot-3 and 130 pounds prior to this, so losing 8 pounds was significant for me. Aside from dropping a few, I also learned that dairy made me feel a bit bloated. It's not that I will never have cheese again, but I try to keep it to a minimum so my tummy is in a happy place.

After your week of almost-torture, you can start to reintroduce foods into your diet again. You will want to do this 1 food at a time, and then give yourself a few days to adjust. This will help you pinpoint any foods that don't exactly agree with your body. I would recommend keeping a food journal to note any differences in energy, sleep, and/or bowel movement (sorry, I know it is gross, but it is necessary).

If you start to notice changes that are less than desirable, you can make note that you may have an intolerance to this type of food and that you need to reduce the amount you consume in your diet after consulting with your doctor. This gives you the power to figure out what foods work for you and which are just not worth your discomfort.

Gimme a Break

Sometimes you just want to have a little cheat. I'm here to tell you that it's ok. It is thought that you can only be either completely ripped or unhealthy. Watching an interview recently of this hot actor that is known for how he can move his hips (you know who I'm talking about?), he was discussing food on the set of a movie he just released with other hot and chiseled male actors. During the entire time they were filming, the actors were on a super-strict boiled chicken and broccoli diet. Not verbatim, but you get the idea. After they wrapped up the final scene for the movie, this super-hot actor that is really good at doing lap dances bought a whole buffet of junk food. I'm talking chips, candy, and fried chicken. You name it. He also proceeded to state how they were all so sick afterward. They were not surprised, but they were grateful they deprived themselves so women across America could have 90 minutes of pure enjoyment in the movie theater. The point is that eating super-strict is not sustainable.

Why does there have to be one or the other? When you picked up this book, I told you that this wasn't a book to build a six-pack. This is a book to help you develop a healthier life. Part of that is enjoying the life you are already living. I am not saying that food is a direct link to happiness, but maybe having a piece of cake on your birthday is something worth having.

Moderation is key. For me, I like to have a few bites of dark chocolate on occasion. Not a candy bar; just a small square of chocolate.

Ghirardelli sells them in tiny squares that I like, or you can just break off a small piece from a larger bar and put the rest in the fridge for later. Make it the good stuff free of fake chocolate and chemicals. I also love homemade pita chips and hummus. I am a sucker for some good chips and salsa. In the evenings, you will also definitely find me unwinding with a delicious glass of red wine. You'll notice that none of these are over the top, but still satisfy me, so I don't feel completely deprived. Now let's talk about you. What are your favorite cheats that keep your cravings at bay?

Things to Remember:

- •. Don't keep the crap in your house. If it's not around, you can't eat it.
- •. Veggies and fruits. Eat them!
- •. If it can last years on a shelf, then it probably shouldn't spend a second on your lips.
- •. Cheat snack or meal is ok. Cheat day? Just say no!
- •. Save money by buying fruits and veggies that are in season. Try new things. You never know what you may like!

~~~~~Quick and Easy~~~~~

Jennifer Hoffman is a 40-something full-time physician, mother, and loving wife. I mentioned earlier that there are some of you out there that are being pulled in 50 different directions. She regularly comes to my boot camp in the park classes as well as running on other days. Sometimes with her 9-year-old daughter biking alongside her as a workout buddy.

Jennifer's life is nothing short of crazy. When chatting with this busy mom of 2 about how she creates healthy meals for her family, she responded, "I loooooove my pressure cooker! I make a full meal of rice, lentils, and veggies in less than 20 minutes." This makes it simple to throw something together after a long day of seeing patients at the hospital. To help her maintain a healthy weight, she also follows a mainly pescatarian diet that is primarily plant-based.

Although eating mostly clean, Jennifer still allows for a little cheat. "My rule at home is one sweet a day to try and teach my daughter moderation." Understanding what an appropriate portion size looks like (not likely what you would get in any restaurant) will help to keep that waistline in check.

~~~~~~

Tasty Eats

You have your healthy foods all stocked up. More fruits and veggies have been making their way into your meals. Now it's time to explore and try a new spin on all of your favorites and some that are completely new to your taste buds. Over the years as a trainer, many of you have come to me saying that you don't have time to cook healthy or that eating healthy is expensive. I get it. Eating healthy can be both time consuming as well as expensive. I'm here to help you minimize both.

When I first started off as a trainer, I had to constantly be at the gym to find clients to build my business, and I had to look healthy so people wanted to work with me. Since I was just building my business, my paychecks were barely letting me get by, and I got home late, leaving me with little energy to cook. Sound familiar? Most people can relate to one or the other. Maybe you relate to both of these.

Studying nutrition over the years so I could remain healthy and help my clients achieve sustainable weight goals has left me with a whole book full of recipes. This is not a meal plan. I hate strict diets, counting calories, or having to eat a certain amount of anything. We've established that time is of the essence, so I have put together meals that are nutritious and quick. The more you get used to putting meals together, the more you will also find ways to use what you have in your house to modify these recipes to fit your needs.

Breakfast

Overnight Oats

These are great to make a few at a time so you have something to grab and go in the morning.

Apple Cinnamon

½ c uncooked oats

½ c milk alternative (almond, cashew, or coconut milk)

½ c apple, chopped

⅛ tsp ground cinnamon

1 tsp honey or agave syrup

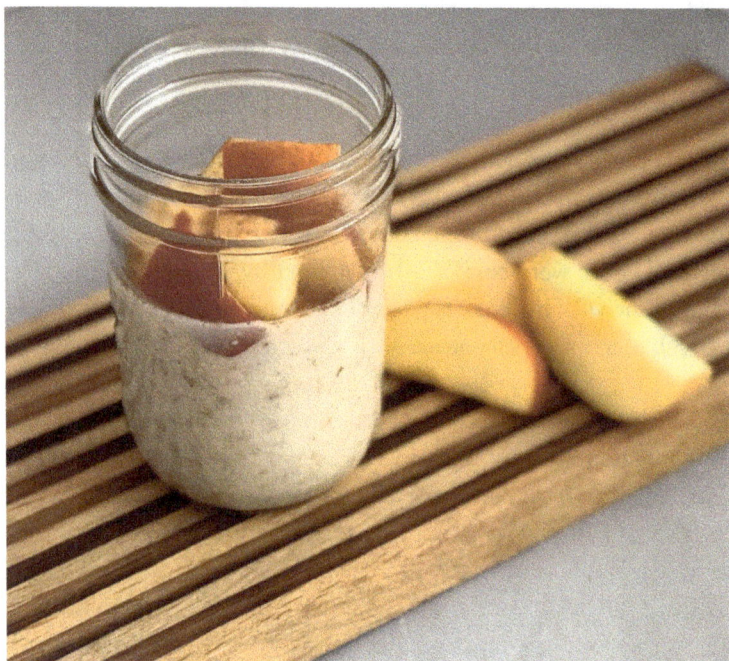

Banana Nut

½ c uncooked oats

1 ripe banana, sliced and smashed

½ c milk alternative (almond, cashew, or coconut milk)

½ tsp ground cinnamon

⅛ tsp nutmeg (optional)

1 tsp honey or agave syrup

¼ tsp vanilla

2 T walnuts, chopped (optional)

Pumpkin Spice

½ c uncooked oats

½ c milk alternative (almond, cashew, or coconut milk)

½ c pumpkin pie filling

2 T walnuts, chopped (optional)

Tip: *1 tsp chia seed can be added to any of these for an extra protein boost.*

Directions:

1. *Add all of the ingredients into a small-size storage container, such as a mason jar.*
2. *Mix together and put in your fridge overnight.*
3. *Enjoy the next morning either cold or warm it up in your microwave! (Only heat up in a microwave-safe container.)*

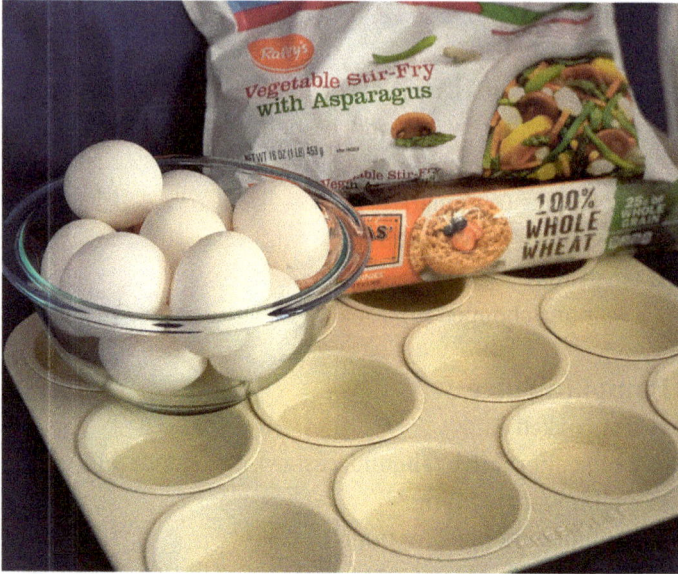

Veggie Breakfast Sandwich

These little egg muffin cups come in handy to throw together a breakfast sandwich in the morning. I recommend making these on a Sunday and just popping the cups in a plastic ziplock bag. Easy to reheat in the microwave and put together in just a few minutes so you can chomp down during your morning commute.

2 c veggies, chopped
10 eggs
Whole wheat English muffins
Muffin pan
¼ avocado per sandwich, sliced (optional)
Sliced Swiss cheese (optional)

Tip: *You really can't go wrong with this. Just pick what you like. Save time by choosing frozen veggie combos that are already chopped. My fave veggie combos:*
• *Spinach, mushroom, and onion*
• *Asparagus, Swiss chard, and green onion*
• *Bell pepper (any color), mushrooms, and cauliflower*

Directions:

1. *Preheat oven to 375°F.*
2. *Grease a muffin pan with non-stick cooking spray, or dab a paper towel in avocado or sunflower oil and lightly coat the pan.*
3. *Chop your veggies. Sauté veggies for a few minutes in a pan with either water, vegetable stock, or 1 tsp of avocado or sunflower oil. Cook for 2 to 3 minutes to where they are starting to soften but not cooked all the way. Harder veggies like asparagus, onions, and cauliflower should cook for the full time. Add in your leafy greens like spinach and chard for the last minute, as they cook quickly.*
4. *While the veggies are cooking, crack all 10 eggs in a large bowl and whisk thoroughly until blended. Let the veggies cool for a few minutes, and then add to egg mixture and stir.*
5. *Pour egg mixture evenly into each muffin cup, and bake for 15 to 17 minutes or until eggs are cooked through.*
6. *Allow eggs to cool for 5 to 10 minutes. In the meantime, toast your English muffin and slice your avocado, if using.*
7. *Assemble your sandwich and enjoy!*

Smoothies

This is your traditional grab-and-go breakfast. Personally, I enjoy these more during the warmer months, but the simplicity of them has many gravitating for these blended drinks year-round. There are so many options, so feel free to make swaps to put your own spin on them. These can be prepped the night before with a quick 30-second blend in the morning before you dash out the door.

Tip: *As bananas become really ripe, you can peel them, break them in half, and put them in a freezer ziplock bag for future smoothie making.*

Green Hawaiian Smoothie

1 handful of spinach
2 c frozen tropical fruit mix (mango, pineapple, etc.)
½ ripe banana
1 c strawberries
1 c milk alternative (almond, cashew, or coconut)
1 tsp chia seed (optional)

Sunny Strawberry Smoothie

1 c strawberries
½ c peaches
1 c milk alternative (almond, cashew, or coconut)
1 tsp chia seed (optional)

PB & J Smoothie

1 c strawberries
½ ripe banana
¼ c natural peanut butter
1 c milk alternative (almond, cashew, or coconut)

Directions:

1. Dump everything in a smoothie blender, like a NutriBullet.
2. Blend thoroughly for 30 seconds to 1 minute.
3. Drink up!

Toast 3 Ways

Toast with butter and jam is so yesterday. Make a meal with your toast so that it is appealing to both your eyes and your stomach. I prefer either Dave's Killer Bread or Ezekiel bread (check the freezer at your grocer), but any whole wheat bread will do. Just read the label to ensure that whole wheat flour is the first ingredient and that there is no high-fructose corn syrup. Who needs sugar in their bread anyway? Gross!

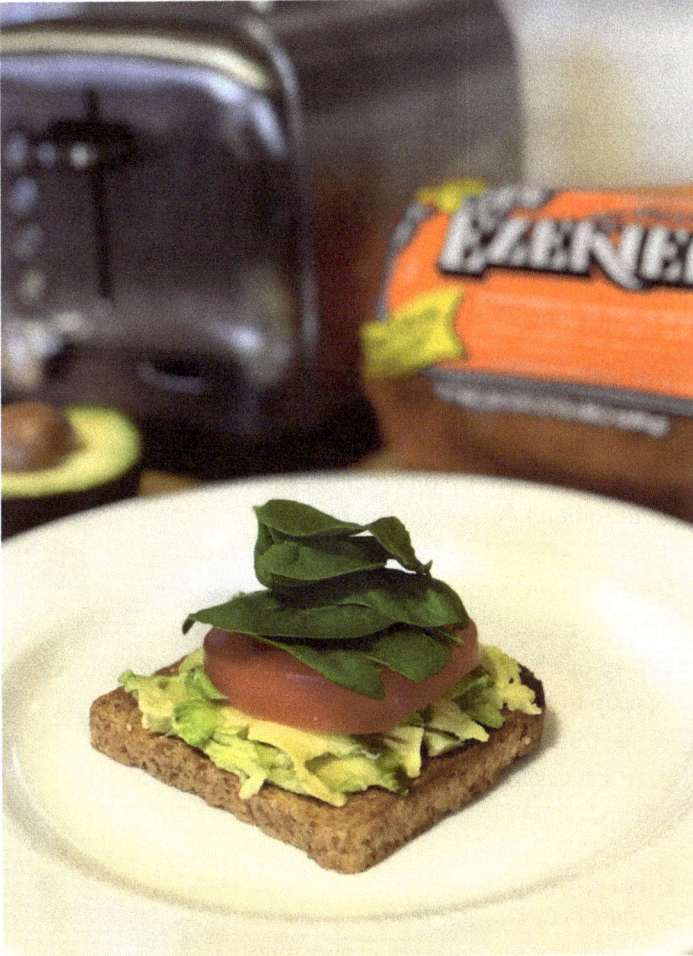

Peanut Butter with Banana

2 slices of whole wheat bread (Dave's Killer Bread or Ezekiel)

1 T natural peanut butter (just peanuts and salt, no sugar)

½ banana, sliced

Ground cinnamon

Directions:

1. Toast bread to your liking.

2. Smear peanut butter.

3. Arrange banana slices (you could make this into a smile for fun).

4. Sprinkle cinnamon, and take a bite.

Avocado with Tomato

2 slices of whole wheat bread (Dave's Killer Bread or Ezekiel)

½ avocado, smashed

½ handful of spinach

1 to 2 slices of tomato

Salt and pepper to taste

Directions:

1. Toast bread to your liking.

2. Spread avocado.

3. Layer with spinach and tomatoes.

4. Add salt and pepper, if you like.

Open-Faced Omelet Sandwich

Ingredients:

2 slices of whole wheat bread (Dave's Killer Bread or Ezekiel)

Egg cup from veggie breakfast sandwich

½ handful of spinach or arugula

¼ avocado, sliced (optional)

Salt and pepper to taste

Directions:

1. Toast bread to your liking.

2. Smash egg cup and spread over toast.

3. Layer greens on top with sliced avocado, if you choose.

4. Salt and pepper to taste.

Lunch

Salad in a Jar

These easy-to-go salads not only look cool but are also an easy way to bring a salad on the go. I would suggest making a few at a time so you have a healthy lunch to grab on your way to work or school, or you could have a light dinner on an evening when you don't feel like cooking.

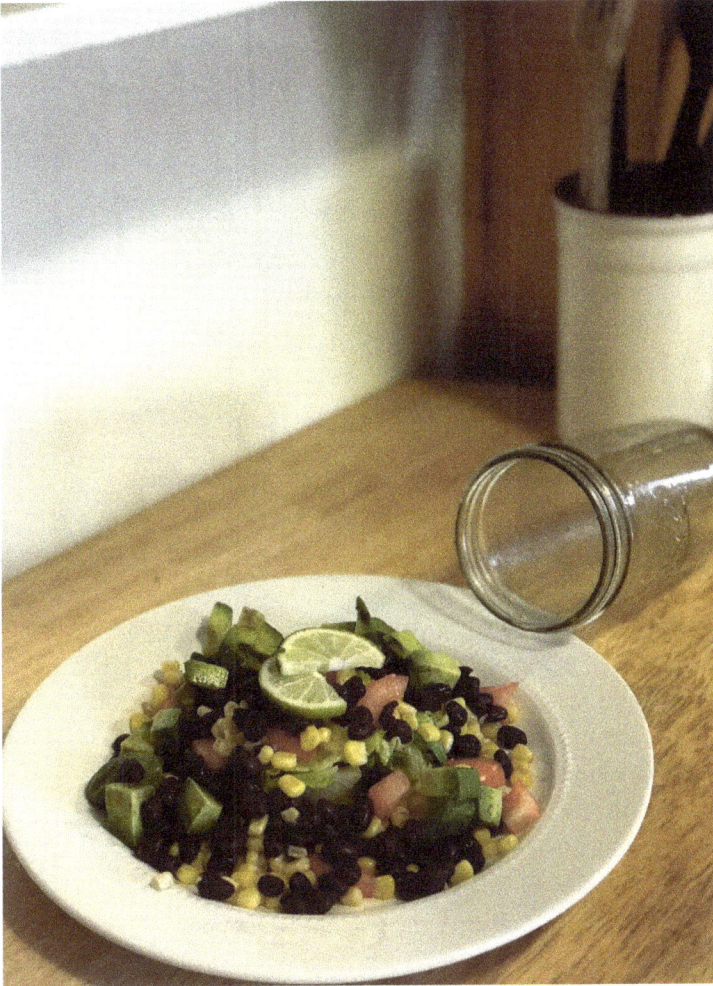

Cabo Fresh

Juice from 1 lime
1 T extra-virgin olive oil
½ avocado, diced
2 T chopped green onion or cilantro
½ c corn, rinsed
1 c black beans, rinsed
½ medium-sized tomato, seeded and chopped
1 to 2 handfuls of lettuce (romaine, spring mix, or baby spinach)

Tip: *The juice from the lime will prevent the avocado from browning, so it is important to put them together.*

Take Me to Santorini

Juice from 1 lemon
1 T extra-virgin olive oil
1 T balsamic vinegar
½ tsp dried oregano
⅛ c black or kalamata olives, sliced
1 c diced tomatoes
½ medium cucumber, diced
¼ red onion, sliced
¼ c crumbled feta cheese
1 to 2 handfuls of romaine or spring mix, chopped

ACV Chef

1 T extra-virgin olive oil
1 T apple cider vinegar (ACV)
1 tsp Italian seasoning
1 handful cherry tomatoes
⅛ c black olives, sliced
½ medium cucumber, diced
½ c sliced carrots
½ c sliced bell peppers
1 boiled egg, sliced or chopped
1 to 2 handfuls of romaine or spinach, chopped

Tip: *ACV has been shown to have many health benefits, such as helping acid reflux, lowering blood pressure, improving diabetes, and supporting weight loss. Use ACV in any recipes calling for regular white vinegar for an extra health kick.*

Directions:

1. *Layer each ingredient in the order listed in a mason jar.*
2. *Seal with the lid and store in your fridge for up to 3 to 5 days.*
3. *Dump directly onto a plate or in a bowl when you are ready to eat.*

Supple Kale and Avocado Salad

This salad I separated from the others as it is best to consume within 24 hours of preparation. However, it is one of my faves, so I couldn't keep it a secret from all of you. If you aren't too sure about kale, please give this a try. To me, massaging the kale makes all the difference!

3 handfuls of kale, chopped
1 T extra-virgin olive oil
Juice from 1 lemon
1 c cooked quinoa
1 handful cherry tomatoes
Salt and pepper to taste
½ avocado, diced

Directions:

1. *In a large bowl, add your kale. Drizzle in the oil and lemon juice on top. With your hands, start to scrunch up the kale. Just take a big handful, and give it a tight squeeze. Continue until the kale starts to soften a bit. You will also notice that it slightly shrinks.*
2. *Add in your quinoa, tomatoes, and salt or pepper. Toss with hands or a utensil.*
3. *Top with avocado.*

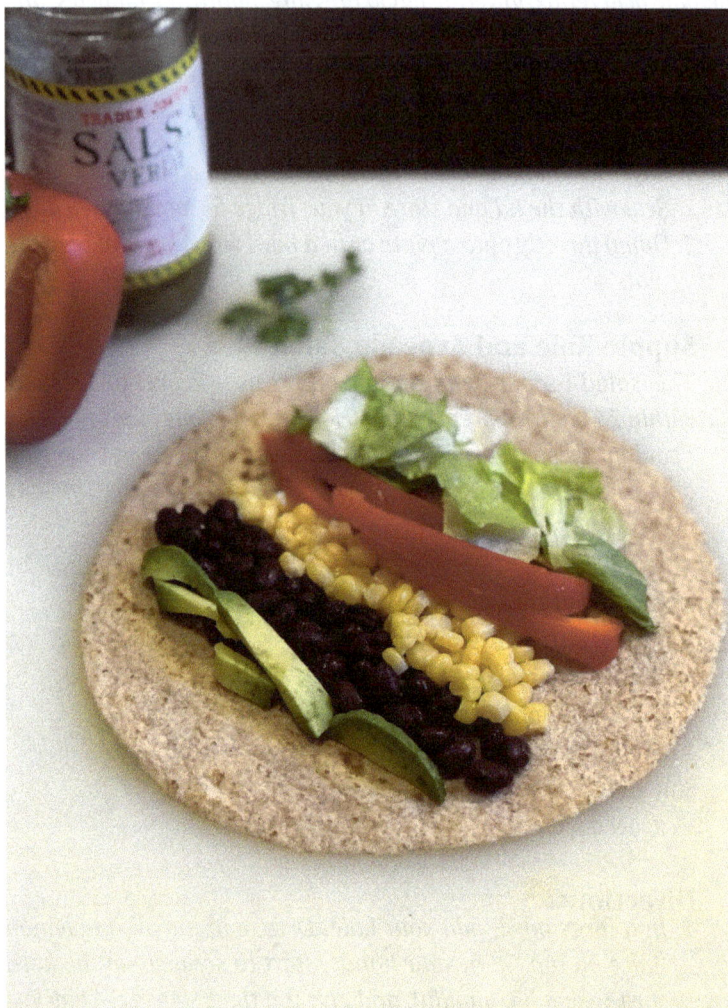

Wraps

These are basically like burritos but with just different ingredients. An easy grab-and-go meal if you are unable to sit down with a plate and fork. Plus, who doesn't love to eat with their hands!

Power Protein Wrap

1 whole wheat or spinach burrito-sized tortilla

¼ c hummus

¼ c sliced beets

1 handful spinach

¼ c cooked quinoa

Mexican Salsa Wrap

1 whole wheat or spinach burrito-sized tortilla

½ c black beans

¼ c corn

¼ c red bell pepper, sliced

1 handful romaine, chopped

2 T of your favorite salsa

¼ avocado, chopped (optional)

Gobble-It-Up Wrap

1 whole wheat or spinach burrito-sized tortilla

4 slices of deli-sliced turkey

¼ tomato, sliced

⅛ c sliced onion

1 handful spinach

¼ avocado, sliced

Tip: *Deli-sliced meat from your deli counter is generally lower in sodium compared to the pre-packaged stuff found in the refrigerated section. With fewer preservatives, your meat will be fresher. Fresh just tastes better!*

Directions:

1. Layer all ingredients in the center of the tortilla.

2. Fold the long end on 1 side about 1/3 of the way.

3. Roll up the tortilla completely and chomp away!

Bowls are kind of like salads minus the lettuce. These will not only fill your belly with so much nutritional goodness, but will also warm you from the inside out. Perfect any time there is a chill in the air!

Rustic Chicken Quinoa Bowl

3 to 6 oz chicken breast

Dash of cayenne (optional)

½ sweet potato, cubed

1 c broccoli

1 c cooked quinoa

Salt and pepper to taste

Directions:

1. *Slice chicken into 1/4-inch slices. Sprinkle with cayenne, if you like extra spice. Sauté in pan until no longer pink.*
2. *Take sweet potato and broccoli and steam until soft (approximately 3 to 6 minutes). I also like to sprinkle my sweet potato with cayenne. For a quicker option, you can also microwave for 2 to 3 minutes.*
3. *Layer quinoa on bottom of bowl.*
4. *Take sweet potato, broccoli, and chicken and place on top.*
5. *Add salt and pepper to taste.*

Edamame Asian Bowl

1 c shredded carrots (you can buy pre-shredded to save time)

1 c shredded red cabbage

1 green onion

1 c brown rice, cooked

1 c cooked edamame (buy frozen and shelled)

1 tsp sesame seeds (optional)

1 T Extra-virgin olive oil

Salt and pepper to taste

Directions:

1. *Shred your carrots and red cabbage if you did not buy pre-shredded.*

2. *Cut the onion root off (the tip on the white end), and then cut in half. Thinly slice the onion longways.*

3. *Layer rice on bottom of bowl. Place carrots, cabbage, and edamame on top.*

4. *Put a pan on low to medium heat. Once warm, place sesame seeds (if using) in pan and toss until toasted, around 1 to 2 minutes. Keep a close eye on them, as they will start to turn brown quickly. Set aside in small bowl.*

5. *Take your olive oil and place in a p jan on low to medium heat. Once the oil is warm, place sliced green onions in for 2 to 3 minutes or until fragrant. Remove from heat, and stir in toasted sesame seeds.. 6 Drizzle olive oil and green onion dressing over bowl. Salt and pepper to taste.*

Time saver: *Many grocers carry pre-cooked rice and sometimes quinoa in the instant rice section. This can save a ton of time, since they generally only take 90 seconds to cook in the microwave.*

Snacks

Pinwheel Bites

These little grab-and-go treats have a mix of carbs and protein to keep you going until your next meal. Make these in advance and keep in the fridge for a convenient and healthy treat.

Hummy In My Tummy

1 whole wheat or spinach burrito-sized tortilla

¼ c hummus

1 handful spinach

½ c bell peppers, chopped

PB & A

1 whole wheat burrito-sized tortilla

3 T natural peanut butter (peanuts and salt only)

½ apple, cored and thinly sliced

1 tsp ground cinnamon

Directions:

1. *Layer each ingredient over the entire tortilla.*
2. *Starting on one end, tightly roll the tortilla.*
3. *Create 1-inch slices and enjoy a few at a time for a midday snack.*

Tahitian Escape

This pineapple salsa is not only great with the pita crisps (see next recipe), but it makes a great topping to grilled chicken, white fish, or pork. It is also full of flavor!

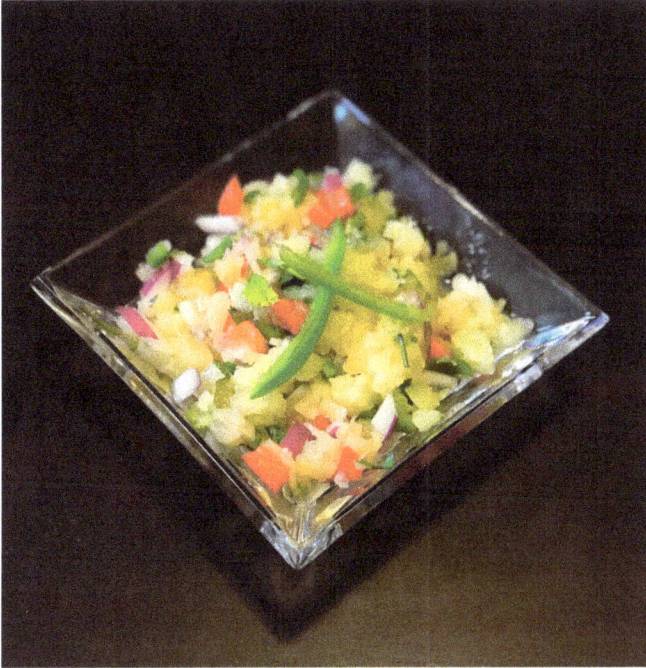

20 oz crushed pineapple

1 red bell pepper, finely chopped

1/2 red onion, finely chopped

½ bunch cilantro, chopped

1 jalapeno, finely chopped

Directions:

1. Mix all of the ingredients into a storage safe container.

2. Place into the fridge, and let the flavors set for a minimum of 6 hours.

3. Enjoy as either a salsa or bake with a lightly flavored protein.

Pita Crisps

Do you like something crunchy but need something healthier than chips? Me too! These are super simple and great for dipping or on their own.

1 whole wheat pita bread
Non-stick cooking spray (preferably olive oil or coconut oil)
Optional seasonings: ground cayenne, ground cinnamon, ground garlic, salt

Directions:

1. *Preheat oven to 400°F.*
2. *Take your pita, and break it in half. If it is not already perforated, then use kitchen shears to cut it in half.*
3. *With your half, cut in half again. Then cut that in half again. Cut everything in half one more time. Repeat for the other half. You should be left with 16 pieces.*
4. *Peel apart the 16 pieces, and you now have 32 pieces.*
5. *Take a cookie sheet and spray the pan with non-stick cooking spray.*
6. *Lay each pita piece on sheet and spray with cooking spray. Sprinkle with desired seasoning.*
7. *Bake for approximately 8 minutes, flipping at the halfway point.*
8. *Use for dipping or enjoy on their own!*

Rosemary Almonds

2 c whole almonds
1 T extra-virgin olive oil
1 T finely chopped rosemary
Salt to taste (optional)
Ground chili pepper flakes (optional)

Directions:

1. Preheat oven to 325°F.
2. Mix all ingredients in a medium-sized bowl.
3. Line a cookie sheet with tin foil and layer almonds.
4. Bake for approximately 20 minutes or until lightly toasted.
5. Let cool, and snack away!

Dinner

Mexico with a Punch of Quinoa

This dish is a must-bake! I have seriously so many requests for this dish, and numerous people that thought they hated quinoa dig in for seconds. I promise this will not disappoint.

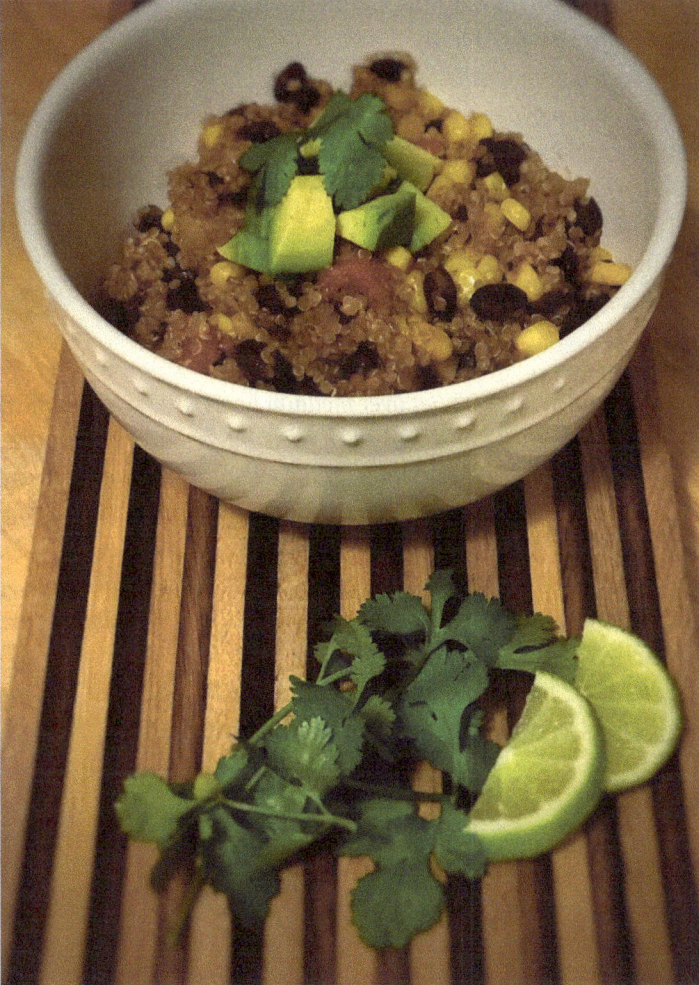

1 T oil (avocado, sunflower, or canola oil)

½ onion, chopped

2 chicken breasts, diced (optional)

2 cloves garlic, minced

1 jalapeno, seeded and minced

1 c uncooked quinoa

1 c vegetable broth

1 15 oz can of black beans, drained and rinsed

1 14.5 oz fire-roasted tomatoes

1 c corn (canned or frozen)

1 tsp chili powder

½ tsp cumin

½ avocado, diced

1 bunch cilantro, chopped

1 lime, quartered

Salt to taste (optional)

Directions:

1. *Heat oil in large skillet over medium heat. After a few minutes, add the onions and cook until fragrant, about 2 to 3 minutes.*
2. *Add the chicken (if adding), and cook until no longer pink.*
3. *Add the garlic and jalapeno until fragrant, about 1 to 2 minutes.*
4. *Add in all of the remaining ingredients except the avocado, cilantro, and lime. Bring to a boil. 5. Reduce to simmer, and cover for 20 minutes.*
6. *Remove from heat and stir. Serve into a bowl, and top with cilantro, avocado, and lime. Salt to taste.*

Bowl Full of Chili

This is my absolute fave for a cold day. It's hearty and is a total comfort food for me. Make it your own by swapping out some of the veggies.

2 T oil (avocado, sunflower, or canola)
1 onion, chopped
1 green bell pepper, diced
2 to 3 garlic cloves, minced
1 lb beef or turkey (optional)
3 cans of beans (can mix it up with kidney, black beans, garbanzo, or chili)
2 14.5 oz cans diced tomatoes
1 15 oz can tomato sauce
8 oz sliced mushrooms
2 to 3 T chili powder
1 T cumin
½ c chopped and pickled jalapeno (optional)
Salt to taste
1 bunch cilantro, chopped

Directions:
1. *Heat oil in large pot for 2 to 3 minutes. Add in onion, bell pepper, and garlic. Stir occasionally until fragrant. Add in beef or turkey if using, and cook until brown.*
2. *Add in all of the remaining ingredients except salt and cilantro.*
3. *Bring to a boil, and then reduce to a simmer. Cover for 30 minutes stirring occasionally.*
4. *Salt to taste.*
5. *Serve in a bowl and top with cilantro if desired.*

Tip: *If you are making this for 1 to 2 people, I would suggest putting half of this into a freezer bag and lying it on a cookie sheet in your freezer to save for a later date. You can do the same thing for soups and stews so that you have a healthy meal to thaw out with little effort.*

Veggie Pasta Bake

Quick, easy, and full of veggies. You can make this while you help the kiddos with their homework or as you savor a glass of wine.

1 lb uncooked rigatoni or fusilli

1 jar pasta sauce

1 c sliced squash (Italian or yellow crookneck)

1 c sliced mushrooms

1 c chopped broccoli

1 c shredded parmesan (optional)

Directions:

1. *Fill a large pot with water and bring to a boil.*
2. *Add pasta for 4 to 5 minutes.*
3. *Preheat oven to 450°F.*
4. *Drain pasta and add back into pot with remaining ingredients except the parmesan.*
5. *Mix and then add to 9x13-inch pan.*
6. *Bake in oven for 20 to 25 minutes. Add the shredded parmesan in the last 5 minutes, if adding.*
7. *Let cool for 3 to 5 minutes before serving.*

Rose Marry My Chicken

This marinade is everything! I always have these ingredients on hand which is why it is an easy go-to. My boyfriend is an inspiration to this dish as I use it to convince him that he needs to marry me if he wants to continue to eat well.

1 c water

⅛ c chopped rosemary

½ c extra-virgin olive oil

1 lemon, juiced

½ lemon, whole

3 to 4 garlic cloves

1 tsp salt

1 lb skinless chicken breast

½ lemon, sliced

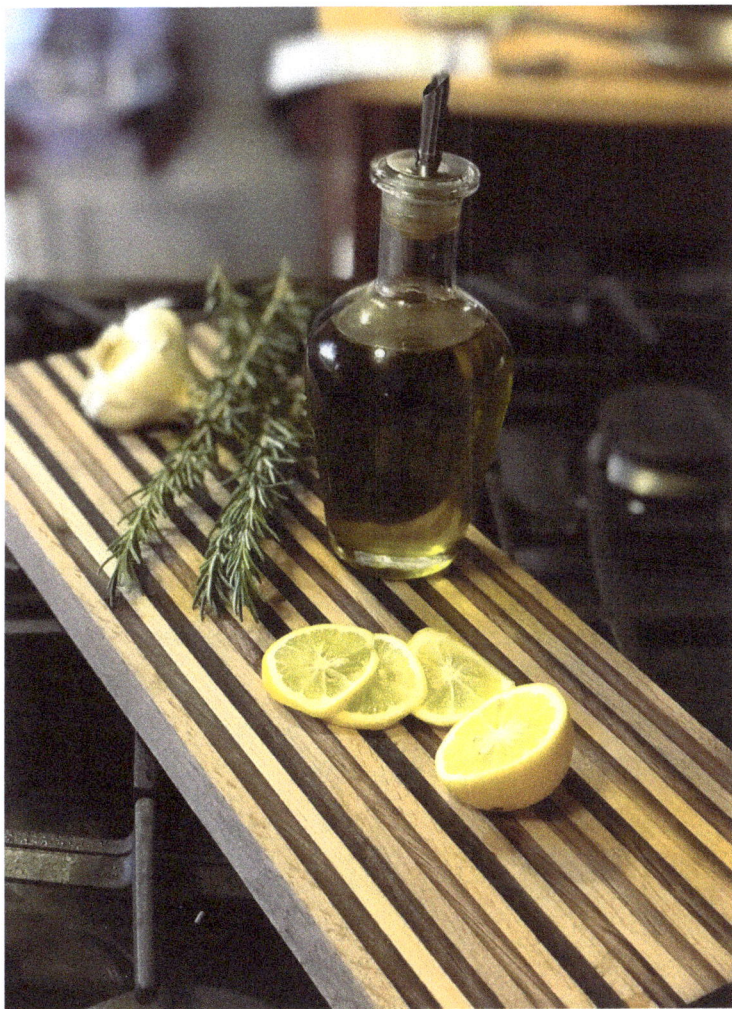

Directions:

1. *Boil water in a small sauce pan. Turn off heat, add rosemary, and cover for 3 to 5 minutes.2.The rosemary will steep like tea, pulling the flavors from the leaves.*

3. *In a food processor or smoothie blender, add all of the ingredients except for the chicken, ½ lemon and lemon slices.*

4. *Blend until all mixed, approximately 30 seconds.*

5. *Add chicken to a glass dish or ziplock storage bag. Pour rosemary and garlic mixture over chicken.*

6. *Let the chicken marinade at least 2 hours or, even better, overnight.*

7. *You can either bake the chicken in the oven at 400°F for 25 minutes (flipping halfway through) or on a grill for 30 minutes (flipping halfway through). When flipping, juice the ½ lemon over all of the chicken to add moisture. Check that the center is no longer pink prior to serving.*

8. *Garnish with lemon slices.*

Slow Cook Big Taste Chicken Tacos

This is the easiest way to make chicken tacos that I have ever learned. We all can find ways to be healthy, and this one is from my dear friend and new mom, Jill Denny. She can cook like a beast and still be the hostess with the mostess. Inspiration comes from everywhere!

1 lb skinless chicken breast

1 jar of your favorite salsa

1 tomato, seeded and diced

1 bunch cilantro, chopped

¼ avocado, diced

Sliced jalapenos

More of your favorite salsa

Whole wheat taco-size tortillas or butter lettuce leafs

Directions:

1. *In a slow cooker, add your chicken and salsa. If the chicken is frozen, place on low for 8 hours. If chicken is thawed, place on low for 6 hours.*

2. *Go to work. Run errands. Play with your kids. Take a nap. Seriously!*

3. *Once chicken is finished in the slow cooker, take 2 forks and shred the meat. It will literally fall apart.*

4. *Build your tacos with whatever toppings you like!*

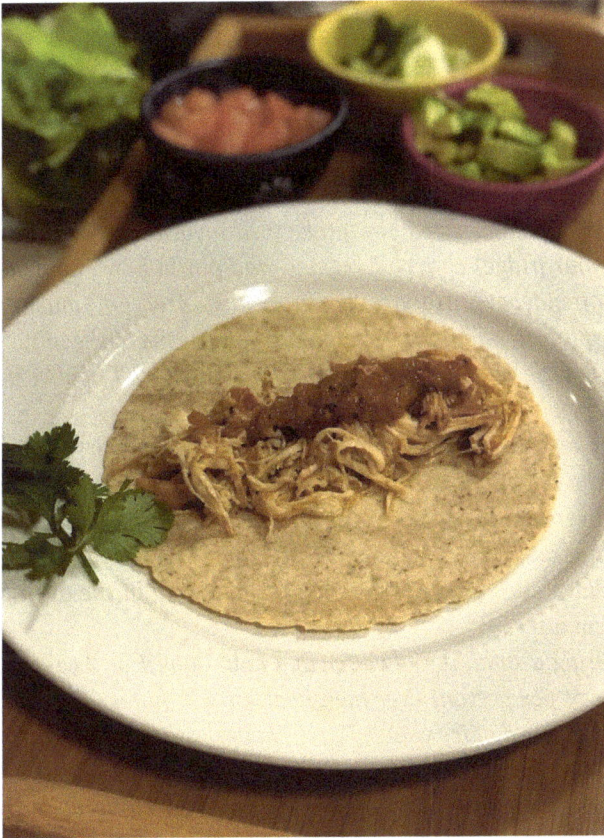

Veggies with Soft-Cooked Eggs

If you like yolk from eggs as gravy, you are not alone. This is a new craving that is sweeping taste buds everywhere. The veggies I put are what I like, but feel free to put in your faves or use up what is in your fridge.

3 to 4 c of your favorite veggies, chopped

1 c beans (butter beans or garbanzo beans)

2 T Extra-virgin olive oil

Salt to taste

2 sheets parchment paper

2 eggs

½ c cooked quinoa

Directions:

1. Heat oven to 400°F.
2. In a medium-sized bowl, take your favorite (or whatever is in your fridge) chopped veggies, and put in bowl. Some repeat offenders I use are green beans, broccoli, mushrooms, spinach, and bell peppers. Add your beans to the mix.
3. Toss the veggie and bean mixture with 1 to 2 T of olive oil and sprinkle with salt.
4. Take 2 sheets of parchment paper and divide the veggie mix to the center of each. Take opposite corners of the paper and fold over several times. Fold up the other ends to seal up the packet.
5. Place each packet on a baking sheet and in the oven for 20 minutes.
6. Bring a small pot of water to a boil. Cook 1 or 2 eggs (cook 1 egg per person) over high heat for 5 minutes. Transfer eggs to a bowl of ice water. Carefully peel the eggs.
7. Once the veggies are cooked, open the packet and stir in the cooked quinoa. Slice open an egg over each packet and watch the yolk ooze out like gravy.
8. Don't drool; just eat!

Reused Stuffed Peppers

It sounds kinda funny, but I am a big believer in saving time in any way possible. This recipe calls for you to reuse your Mexican Quinoa (provided earlier under dinner recipes) and transform it to create a whole new dish. Boom!

1 to 2 red bell peppers

1 c of Mexico with a Punch of Quinoa

⅛ c cheddar cheese (optional)

Directions:

1. Preheat oven to 425°F.

2. Cut off tops of bell peppers. Clean out any seeds on the inside.

3. Place bell pepper upside down on a plate and put on medium-heat in microwave for approximately 3 minutes or until pepper is soft.

4. Stuff quinoa mixture in pepper and top with cheese, if adding. Bake in water-filled (about ½ inch of water) baking sheet for 5 to 10 minutes or until top is crispy.

5. Let cool for 2 to 3 minutes.

Salmon & Veggie Bake

When I was first a personal trainer, this was totally my go-to dinner. No dirty dishes. Will keep you feeling satisfied. Make it even easier by getting the individual salmon pieces at Costco so you can always pull one out to thaw the day of.

1 1/2 T extra-virgin olive oil

Aluminum foil

1 salmon filet

1 T garlic salt

2 c of your fave veggies (asparagus, squash, and mushrooms are my go-tos for this)

1 c cooked brown rice (instant or microwaveable rice to save time)

Salt to taste

Directions:

1. Heat oven to high broil.
2. Smear ½ T olive oil on aluminum foil.
3. Place salmon on center of foil. Season with garlic salt.
4. Lay veggies alongside the salmon. Drizzle remaining oil on veggies and lightly salt. Fold the foil in half and roll up to seal.
5. Roll the open ends to completely seal up the package.
6. Place on a cookie sheet and in oven.
7. Bake for 17 to 19 minutes or until salmon is fully cooked (will be light pink throughout with no dark pink remaining).
8. You can either eat out of the foil to avoid doing dishes or transfer to a plate.

Sides

Fresh Summer Salad
This is always a great accompaniment to any summer BBQ or on its own if you just want something light and fresh.

1 cucumber, chopped

2 tomatoes, seeded and chopped or 2 c halved cherry tomatoes

1 avocado, diced

1 lemon, juiced

1 T extra-virgin olive oil

½ c chopped basil

Salt to taste

Directions:
1. Toss everything in a large bowl.
2. Eat!

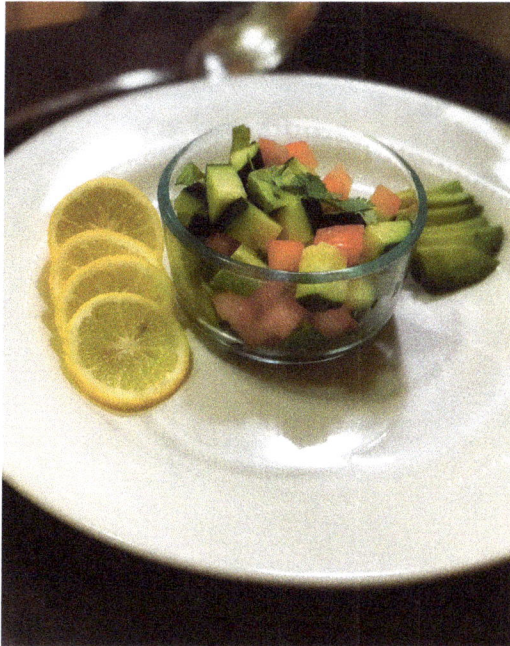

Roasted Veggie Medley

The first time I made this, it was for my southern family that only knew of veggies as deep-fried or from a can. They were pretty convinced that they would not like these Brussels. Not to brag, but there were no leftovers and everyone was asking for the recipe. As you will see, it is about as simple as it gets.

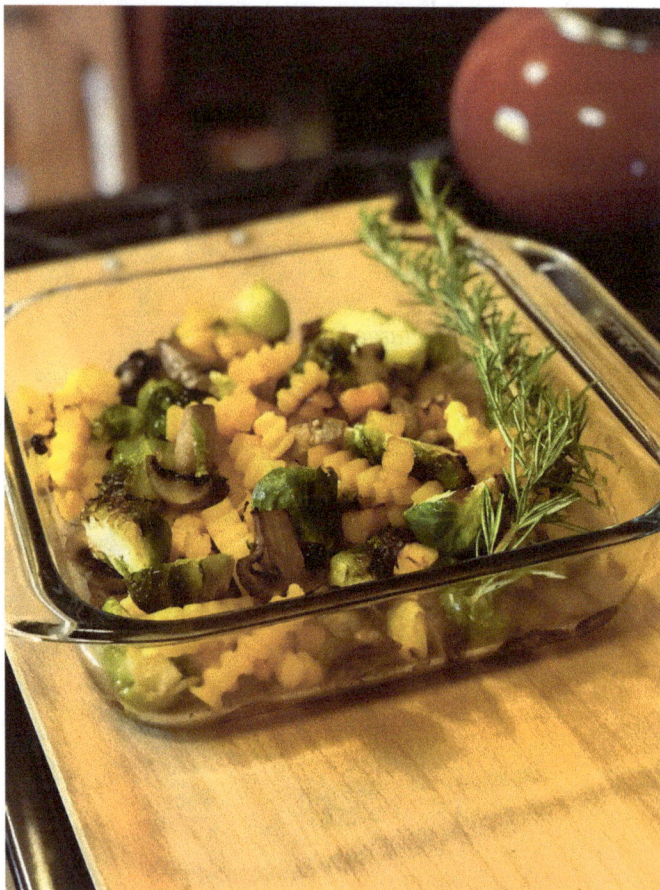

1 lb Brussels sprouts, halved

8 oz mushrooms, quartered or sliced

4 c diced butternut squash

2 T extra-virgin olive oil

Salt to taste

Directions:

1. Preheat oven to 400°F.

2. Toss all of the veggies in a large bowl with the olive oil to coat.

3. Spread on cookie sheet or in 9x13–inch baking dish.

4. Bake in oven for 30 to 40 minutes, tossing the veggies every 10 minutes.

5. Sprinkle with salt after removing from the oven.

6. Let cool for 5 minutes before serving.

Sweet Potato Medallions

You can slice these up like french fries or medallions if you are in a hurry. Either way, they can deliver that sweet, salty, or spicy taste you crave.

1 sweet potato, sliced in medallions or like french fries

1 T extra-virgin olive oil

Seasonings: ground cayenne, ground cinnamon, truffle salt, or regular salt

Directions:

1. Preheat oven to 425°F.

2. Take cut sweet potato and toss with olive oil and desired seasonings.

3. Spread on to cookie sheet and cook for 20 to 25 minutes or until crisp.

4. Let cool for 2 to 3 minutes before serving.

Roasted Asparagus with Balsamic Syrup
So it's obviously not syrup, or it wouldn't be in my book. However, the richness you can draw from balsamic vinegar is so delightful it will seem like an amazing drizzle of bliss. This is the perfect side to any protein.

1 T extra-virgin olive oil
1 bunch of asparagus, trimmed
1 c balsamic vinegar
Salt to taste

Directions:
1. Heat oil on medium heat in pan large enough to fit asparagus.
2. Add asparagus and cook for 8 to 10 minutes until soft yet still firm.
3. Set aside asparagus on plate.
4. Heat same pan to medium/high heat.
5. Add balsamic vinegar and bring to a boil. Reduce to a simmer and cover for 10 minutes.
6. Let cool for 2 to 3 minutes.
7. Drizzle balsamic vinegar over asparagus. Add salt to taste.

Tip: *The balsamic vinegar also makes a great drizzle for a caprese salad over sliced tomatoes, mozzarella, and basil.*

The Other White Veggie
You can choose to add the garlic to this or not, but I love garlic, so obviously, I added it in. It is your choice. I only had cauliflower raw and with ranch dressing until about age 30. It is so much better baked. Just try it!

1 head of cauliflower, chopped
4 to 5 cloves of garlic
3 to 4 T extra-virgin olive oil
Salt to taste

Directions:

1. *Preheat oven to 425°F.*
2. *Toss cauliflower, garlic, and oil in large bowl. Spread on cookie sheet or 9x13-inch baking dish.*
3. *Bake in oven for 35 to 40 minutes. Toss about every 10 minutes.*
4. *Salt to taste once cooked.*

Dessert

Crustless Peach Cobbler

Peach is one of my favorite fruits, but with a buttery crust, it leaves me feeling gross. Enjoy all of the flavors with a lot less of the guilt. Bonus: Your pants fit the next morning.

1 peach, pitted and halved

½ c mascarpone

2 T chopped mint

1 T honey(optional)

Directions:

1. *Take each peach half and grill on either a grill pan on medium/high heat, electric grill, or outside grill (lightly spread olive oil on flesh part of peach if cooking on grill). Cook for 3 to 5 minutes or until golden brown.*
2. *Let peach halves cool for 2 to 3 minutes.*
3. *Top with mascarpone, mint and honey.*

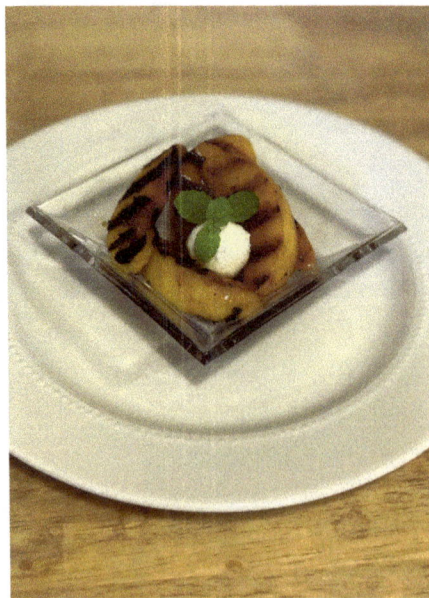

Chocolate Swirl
This recipe is a great use of bananas that go bad. Just peel them and stick them in a freezer ziplock bag. Pull them out to make this icy treat.

1 frozen banana, quartered
2 to 3 tsp cocoa powder
¾ c milk alternative (almond or soy)
½ c ice
Extra: 2 T peanut butter

Directions:
1. Mix all of the ingredients in a blender or blender jar such as a NutriBullet.
2. Scoop out into a glass and treat yourself.

Berry Good Martini
Make this one as treat for yourself, or it even makes a great treat for your dinner party. Lots of nutrition and zero guilt.

1 c plain Greek yogurt
3 strawberries, sliced
⅛ c blueberries
1 T sliced almonds
1 tsp honey

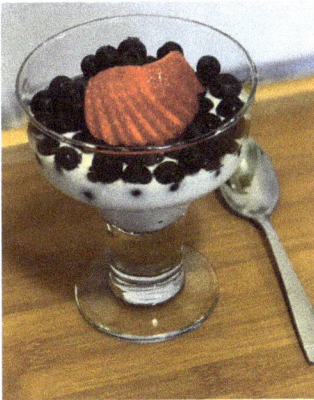

Directions:
1.Layer all ingredients in the order listed in a glass, such as a martini glass.
2. Enjoy!

Pumpkin Oat Cookie Bites

One dessert that was a favorite of mine as a kid was cookies. I craved the perfect cookie! So perfect in fact that after I took a bite of one, it no longer held to my standards of what an ideal cookie looked like. Yes, Princess Christine did not eat broken cookies. These, however, you will want to enjoy down to the very last bite.

2 ½ c oats

1 c pumpkin pie filling

2 to 3 T honey

½ tsp vanilla extract

Extras: ½ c walnuts (chopped), dark chocolate chips, or dried cranberries

Directions:

1. *Preheat oven to 350°F. Spray a cookie sheet with non-stick cooking spray.*
2. *Dump all of the ingredients in a bowl and mix until combined.*
3. *Spoon out and form 15 to 20 balls and place on your cookie sheet.*
4. *Bake for 8 to 10 minutes.*
5. *Let the cookies cool for 5 minutes before removing and pairing with coffee or tea.*

Drinks

Water is something that we know we need to drink a ton of every day, but honestly, it is not always appealing to me. To make things look a bit more enticing, I like to create water that has more color and flavor. Here are the ones that I find myself going back to over and over again.

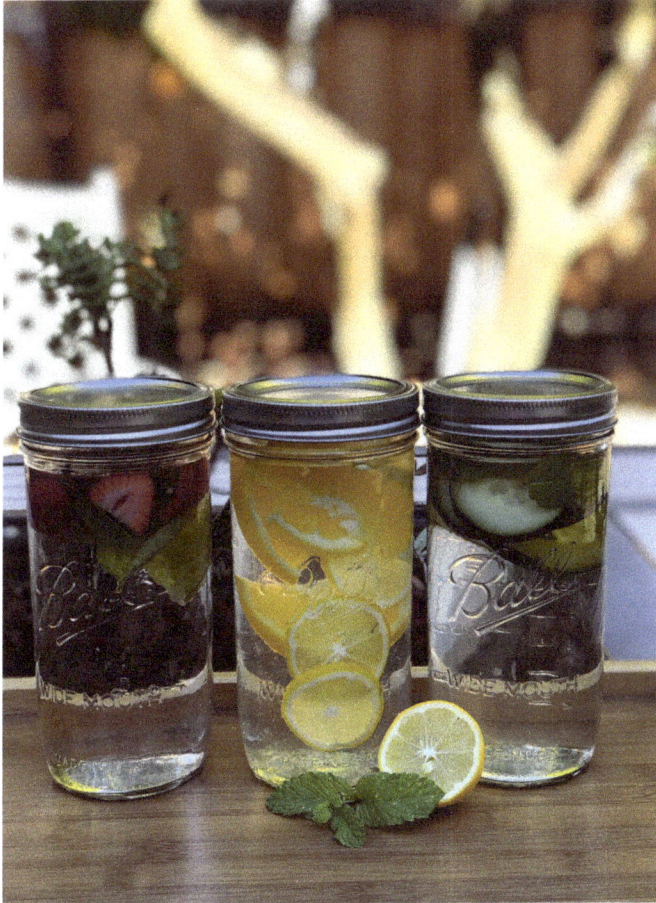

Strawberry-Basil

3 to 5 strawberries, sliced

2 to 3 basil leaves

Cucumber-Mint

⅛ medium-sized cucumber, sliced

1 handful of mint

Orange-Lemon

½ orange, sliced

½ lemon, sliced

Directions:

1. *Add ingredients to refillable water container with a wide-mouth to insert item*
2. *Refrigerate for at least 3 hours and sip away!*

Part 3:

Adding Movement

Starting a fitness routine is tough. Like, really tough. Luckily, it is not an impossible task. You just need to find a way to get the ball rolling. If you go back to the front of your journal that you started as you began reading this book, you will find your why. Those things

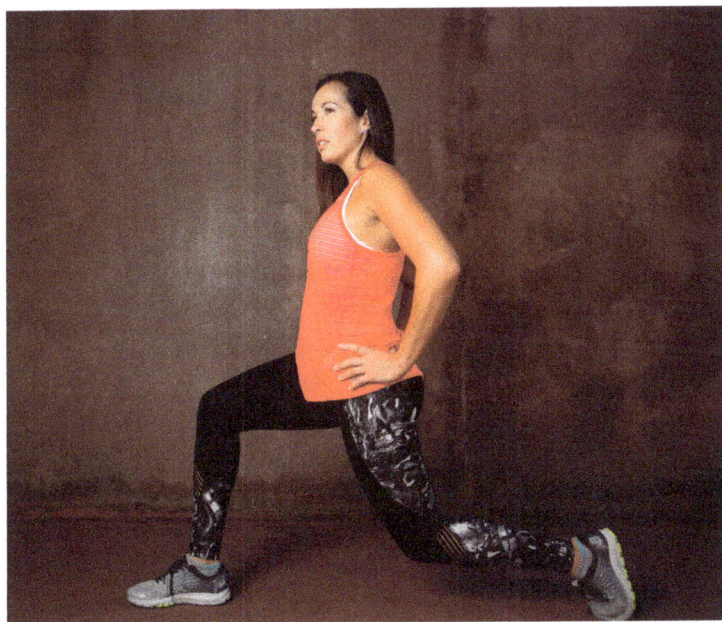

and those people that are so dear to your heart are the very reasons why you are doing this. Partly for yourself, but maybe also so you can remain as a support to others. When you look at your Board of Reason, you have this daily reminder as to why you continue to move forward. The goal is not to be perfect but just to find ways to can sprinkle fitness into your day.

A Schedule
That Works

Just like with your food, planning is a big part of your success in making sure you get in your exercise. It doesn't have to take a lot of time. As a matter of fact, once you build it into your schedule, it should be a part of your day that happens naturally. There will be times that you have so many bumps in the road that getting in your workout just doesn't happen. Don't freak out. You won't gain 100 pounds by skipping a workout here and there. You will gain the weight back, though, if you allow yourself to skip on a regular basis. Let this be the exception.

To find something that works for you, it is important to take a look at your schedule. If yours is anything like mine, it feels completely full until you look at it on paper (or maybe on your fancy smartphone). How do you think I found time to write a book while I am running a 50 to 60 hours a week health and wellness business? You can make the time in your day. A 1-hour workout is only 3% of your day. If you are starting from scratch, getting in a few workouts in a week will equate next to nothing. Think about the times that you are just sitting around figuring out what you're going to do. I'll tell you what you can do in that time. Move your body!

~~~~~ Time to Take a Look ~~~~~

Grab your schedule and sit down with a highlighter. If you don't have your daily tasks listed along with your work schedule, you can download one for free online: Just Google "free weekly calendar." After you have filled in all of your time that is dedicated to things such as going to work, picking up the kids from school, attending church, and making dinner, you will see pockets of remaining time. Woohoo! You actually do have time!

Now is the time to grab that highlighter. Take a look at your schedule and highlight the moments in your day that you have 30 to 45 minutes available. That amount is not a huge time commitment, but you have just identified times you can sprinkle fitness into your life. Now that you have recognized that it is possible to add fitness to your life, list the days and times below, starting with Monday:

1. _____

2. _____

3. _____

4. _____

5. _____

Anytime I am helping a client find time in their week, I always have them front-load their schedule. What does this mean? It means that you will want to plan your workouts earlier in the week as often as possible. The reason for this is that it gives you a bit of a cushion, should something come up. You will have setbacks, and life will not be perfect, but you can still set yourself up for success. The goal here is to find time to sweat a bit and yet have time to go out and enjoy the other things in life. For most of us, this happens Friday through

Sunday. If your workouts are done, then you can feel free to go out and play without any guilt.

~~~~~~~

Deciding When to Start

So now that you know when you have time to exercise, you have to decide when you to get started. Why not now? It seems really ridiculous to me when I hear people say, "I'm going to start getting healthy just as soon as things slow down at work" or "I'm going to start eating healthier after the holidays have passed" or "I'm going to start living a healthy lifestyle blah, blah, blah". I'm here to tell you that there is never going to be a good time to get started.

Don't Be a Stiff Tin Man

We spend so much time sitting: Sitting as we drive to work; sitting when we get to work; sitting to drive back home; sitting to eat dinner; and then sitting to watch TV before we go to bed. All that being sedentary will have your joints feeling stiff and achy. Eventually, you will have tight hip flexors and a weak lower back.

Here are 7 Good Reasons to Get Off Your Tush:
1. It improves mental alertness.
2. It enhances circulation.
3. It reduces muscle tension.
4. It improves focus and concentration.
5. It improves sleep quality.
6. It relieves stress.
7. It eases muscle pain.

It will always feel like work, kids, school, and/or life is just not quite aligned with you starting a new healthy lifestyle. This is not about a complete overhaul. This is about just "sprinkling" exercise into your life. It may look like you are just walking around the field while your kids play soccer. Maybe you start biking to and from work that is 10 to 15 minutes from your house a few times a week. You might also find yourself doing the exercises in this section on your lunch break between client meetings. Trust me when I say the little things will add up. More importantly, you will start to feel good inside about doing something healthy for yourself. The bottom line: Start today!

Buddy Up

As motivated as you may be now, there will be times that you will feel completely overwhelmed, tired, or just bored. It's rarely like that in the beginning. Think about a gym at the start of the New Year. Everyone there wants to workout, to get into shape, and they are excited about doing something good for themselves again. Fast forward to March of the same year. Where the heck did everyone go? Accountability is such a huge factor in long-term success. Unless you are a highly motivated person that just loves fitness and works out constantly (for the record, I do not fit into this category even though I am a trainer), you will likely start to skip your workouts to attend happy hour, binge watch the new season of whichever show, or just to surf the internet.

There are several ways to create accountability. My favorite way is to find a workout partner. This could be someone else that is already physically active, or maybe it is someone that wants to be. There are also apps like Dietbet or Gym-Pact that have a group of people that want to be healthier like you but with money on the line. Talk about move it or lose it! If you have a good network of supportive friends and family on social media, you can also proclaim your goals for added support. Just putting it out there with occasional updates makes it feel real. You never know when you may inspire someone in your direct circle that wants to join you to create their own health journey.

Pump It Up or Run It Out?

Aaahhhhhh ... the big debate on whether or not you should focus on lifting weights or doing cardio. Here's the truth; both are important. It's just like your diet. If all you ate was broccoli and spinach, would you be healthy? Of course not! While broccoli and spinach are very healthy for you, other foods provide vital nutrients to you that broccoli and spinach don't have.

Exercise is no different. If all you did was run, then you would be missing out on strengthening your upper body as well as the muscles that help you move from side to side and back to front. On the other hand, if you just lift weights with long breaks in between, then you would miss out on building endurance to go up a flight of stairs without becoming breathless.

Round It Out

Most people either favor cardio or strength training over the other. That is ok. My preference is lifting weights over cardio. There are very few cardio exercises that I actually enjoy. Again, I know I am a personal trainer, and I am supposed to love working out, but that's not the case. I like how I feel after I workout. I also like looking at my Board of Reason knowing that I am taking care of myself for people other than me.

So what's the best type of cardio? The best cardio for you is the one that you enjoy doing. Sure going for a run or taking a spin class will torch major calories, but if you absolutely dread putting on your running shoes, how long do you really think you will keep doing it? Remember when I talked about those New Year's resolutioners? There's your answer. It won't last long if you can't find some fun in your exercise. Regardless of what burns more calories, it will burn more than if you do nothing at all.

To start, I want to you incorporate 3 active days into your schedule. When you went through your availability, you were able to find 3 to 5 timeslots to dedicate to exercise. Now choose your preferred type of exercise and write it in for 2 days. On the third day, write in your not so favorite. It's about balance, remember.

Getting Your Heart Pump On

The thing that makes me curl into a tiny little ball and curdle? Cardio. Ugh! As a female, I am supposedly supposed to love this format of workout over anything in the world. They even have a term for it. Cardio Queen! Honestly, it totally repulses me to think about it, but I know that this form of exercise is important. Sometimes you don't want to hear the truth, but science is science.

According to a study conducted by the Mayo Clinic, here are my favorite top 6 reasons for including aerobic exercise into your fitness routine:

1. **Maintain a healthy weight:** Combined with a healthy diet, cardio can help you lose weight and keep it off.

2. **Improved stamina:** After a consistent cardio plan is established, you will have noticeable results of reduced fatigue and an increase in stamina.

3. **Get sick less often:** Cardiovascular exercise helps to support the immune system leaving you with less sick days and more days to do things you enjoy.

4. **Lower your health risk:** Heart pumping exercises can drop your risks of obesity, heart disease, high blood pressure, type 2 diabetes, stroke, and certain cancers.

5. **Clear the arterial pipes:** Getting your sweat on can help boost your good cholesterol (HDL) and reduce your bad cholesterol (LDL) resulting in less plaque along the arterial walls.

6. **More feel-good hormones:** Get your endorphin high and you will notice your mood improve. Exercise also assists in relaxation and can provide a better night's sleep.

~~~~~*Fit First Principles*~~~~~

As a military veteran and current business consultant, Steve Hussey had to redefine what it meant for him to incorporate exercise back into his life. During his military life physical fitness was integrated into the job description, but then post-military, Steve found himself getting lax about his health. As the years passed, he realized through personal exploration that he wanted to be fit for very specific reasons.

With careful consideration, he realized that the following 3 things were what gave him the most motivation for fusing exercise into his regular lifestyle:

1. To be healthy.
2. To be happy in whatever state his life was in.
3. To be able to do whatever it is he wanted to do physically.

"There are countless studies that show how being fit promotes good health. So having a focus on being and staying fit gives me some personal control over my state of health. As a result, my fitness activity helps me to be happy and see the positive side of things in my personal circumstances, whatever they may be at the time."

A personal accomplishment for Steve occurred after beginning a consistent fitness routine. "I had raced in my earlier years with Sports Car Club of America (SCCA), and I had won two National Championships overall and two other National Championships in my particular class of cars. After more than a decade of not racing, I decided I wanted to return to the sport and be competitive again at the National Championship level.

"While many are not aware, driving an enclosed cockpit sports car in the heat of the summer is a very physically demanding task. So for me, training to improve my upper-body strength and cardio worked really well, and I finished third out of 25 cars in my first year back." Truly, incorporating exercises to improve Steve's overall strength and stamina brought him back to a level of health for his body as well as his mind.

Pumping Iron

So we've established the fact that lifting weights is a good thing. Will you bulk up? It depends on how you lift. Women have a significantly less amount of testosterone than men in order to pack on the muscle. However, this book is not about bodybuilding or getting ripped (remember my "no six-pack" creed?). This is a beginner's guide to getting started, and the first step in doing so is to start strength training.

Building stronger muscles will not only let you do everyday things like carrying in the groceries and grab your Amazon delivery with a bit more ease, but it helps you to do things that you don't even think about. It increases your basal metabolic rate (BMR), which increases the number of calories you burn at rest. That sounds nice, right? Getting to burn calories without having to do anything? It will also help you by providing better support to your joints, which reduces your chances of injury to the major ones, such as your shoulders, hips, and knees. Want to feel like you are 30 when you are 80? You need to improve and maintain your muscle strength for the long haul.

Exercise guidelines are included alongside the workouts I have provided. What you will see are higher rep counts versus using super high weights with a low rep count. You know those guys in the gym that lift up a ridiculous amount of weight and yell like they are the next King Kong? Yeah, that's not going to be us. I mean seriously?!?!? Is that even necessary? Our goal here is for longevity, not to test the limits of our lower back strength and shoulder stability. You just want to start to feel good in your body, am I right? As you will see, the workouts that I have created will focus on completing 15 to 20 reps of each exercise with an emphasis on good form. This will help you to build strength as well as lean muscle.

Bigger Bang for Your Buck

I mentioned earlier how I am not a fan of cardio, right? I am not saying that I am convinced it is not good for you. Broccoli is good for you, but if you don't like it, then you just don't like it. When I started getting into fitness, I thought that there must be a way to make such monotonous movements a little more enjoyable.

When you think about what cardio really is, it is all about getting your heart rate up for an extended period of time. So why does this have to look like running, or biking, or being on an elliptical? I enjoy lifting weights because it makes me feel strong. As women, we are oftentimes looked upon as weak and without muscle. To me, it is empowering to be able to lift a heavy box or move furniture around the house all on my own.

When you begin lifting weights, you will notice that your heart rate will start to increase as well as your body temperature. Instead of taking breaks between exercises, what if you kept your heart beating by moving on to the next exercise with little to no rest? Would you consider that cardio? You bet your ass it is! This is such a major time-saver!

Many times, I am so busy with back-to-back clients that I would have only 2 hours to workout, shower, eat, and be ready for my next client. All you and I need is 30 minutes. That's it! The people that spend 2 to 3 hours in the gym are also doing a lot of chatting with fellow gym members, waiting around for machines, and sitting in the steam room. If you have the time to go workout and hang at the gym, then that is great. My guess is that if you picked up this book, you are looking just to squeeze exercise into your schedule. Squeeze so hard like getting at that last bit of toothpaste left in your tube. As long as it is effective, the quicker, the better.

There are workouts listed in this book. Here's a sample of a strength-training session gone cardio can look:

All for 1 minute each with 20 seconds between

Warm-up
Jumping Jacks
Body-Weight Squats
Cross Punches

Workout
Squats
Push-Ups
Side Lunges
Plank
Back Extensions

Rest 1 minute then repeat workout 4 times

All done!

Big-Boned? Lift to Get Lean

I'm going to get straight to the point. The theory of being big-boned is complete and utter bullshit. I think it is an excuse for people to be heavyset. With that said, we are not all built the same. We come in all different shapes and sizes, and a lot of our body is determined by hormones and genetics.

There are not any legit studies that support the idea of being big-boned. If you feel this is you, have a serious talk with yourself, and ask if you have honestly been living your best life possible with nutrition and exercise. Probably not, and that is totally ok. I just want you to stop making excuses as to why you aren't healthy. We aren't all meant to be a size 0, nor should we be.

Something I don't want you to think, though, is that you are predisposed to your physical condition because of your family members. You can take the reins and seriously overhaul your life. I am sheer proof of this. It is my thought that while some may have to fight harder to achieve a healthy weight, that it is not impossible based on your family's condition. I say this with a heavy heart, but all of my immediate family is either overweight or obese. They eat a diet full of simple carbs, sugar, soda, and a ton of meat, dairy, and processed foods. Exercise is a rare part of their lifestyle, and prescription medications are the norm. I am nowhere near this bad because I find ways to balance my health with nutrition and exercise. I refuse to allow myself to let my body go. I choose to fight to live well while I am alive. Know that you have this same choice.

If you want to lean out, you need to do strength training. You can eventually lift weights, but if you aren't doing anything, then you need to start by just moving your body. Commonly misinterpreted, as you begin to build lean muscle, you will start to lose fat. Fat does not transform to muscle but more so that if you build muscle, you will burn off excess fat. When you do this, you will start to see the shape of your muscles, and you will not only feel strong but look strong too.

Fat requires far less calorie consumption than muscle. Maybe that's why you hear the terms "fat" and "lazy" together. However, most people don't make an adjustment to their caloric intake to accommodate their reduced calorie need. Therefore your body starts to store your excess calories as fat. Not the goal. Can you do strength training exercises to increase your metabolism and allow your body to release fat? Yeeesssss, you can!!!

Bangin' Magical Rearend (BMR)

Ok, so BMR actually has nothing to do with your bootay, but it perked your attention, right? Your basal metabolic rate (BMR) is just in reference to how many calories your body burns at a baseline based on your current activity level, weight, and gender. All you ladies out there don't get sad, but the men will always burn more calories than us. Their typical genetic makeup allows them to build and maintain more muscle than us women can. With that said, it just means that most women would have to work extra hard to achieve similar levels. All this means is that you don't need to match your man at the dinner table. Be mindful of your needs, and just be ok with it. It is about asking for the support of your partner to not pressure you into eating more than you need or guilt you into eating or not eating something.

I have personally been in relationships where my significant other pressured me to eat foods that I knew were not good for me. Potato chips, ice cream, pizza, you name it. Sometimes I think that people who know that have not quite committed to a healthier lifestyle project their lack of control on those around them that are trying to be healthy. It's kind of like getting a workout buddy. It's helpful to have someone by your side to guide you to get in your workouts. If you have someone eating total junk with you, then it somehow becomes an easier reality to swallow.

Know that to get to the stage where you just have to maintain a healthy weight you will have to be consistent with a balanced diet and exercise. I promise you it is not as hard to maintain once you are there. When you lay down that solid foundation with lean muscle mass to have a manageable BMR (not the booty but the metabolic one), your body will be able to sustain a certain shape for a while. Even when you fall off the wagon and gain 5 to 10 pounds, you will find it easier to get your butt in gear and put in a good 30 days of hard work to get you back to your happy zone.

I am not really into counting calories. As we reviewed nutrition earlier, I like to focus on more of what you are eating rather than nickel-and-diming every calorie. However, if you are someone who really needs to know where your baseline is and likes math, here you go:

Women: BMR = 655 + (4.35 x [weight, in pounds]) + (4.7 x [height, in inches]) - (4.7 x [age, in years])

Men: BMR = 66 + (6.23 x [weight, in pounds]) + (12.7 x [height, in inches]) - (6.8 x [age, in years])

Once you have calculated this number, you will want to take into account your daily activity level. This, of course, doesn't account for your body composition. If you have more muscle, you will likely be burning calories at a slightly higher rate and vice versa.

Harris Benedict Formula
Take your BMR and multiply it by the appropriate activity factor, as follows:
- •. If you are sedentary (little or no exercise): Calorie calculation = BMR x 1.2
- •. If you are lightly active (light exercise/sports 1 to 3 days per week): Calorie calculation = BMR x 1.375
- •. If you are moderately active (moderate exercise/sports 3 to 5 days per week): Calorie calculation = BMR x 1.55
- •. If you are very active (hard exercise/sports 6 to 7 days per week): Calorie calculation = BMR x 1.725
- •. If you are extremely active (very hard exercise/sports and a physical job or 2x training): Calorie calculation = BMR x 1.9

What Did You Say?

So you have your workout buddy, and you are out on your cardio day. You are both chitchatting about The Game of Thrones finale or the crap your husband tries to pull or the latest tweet about some political figure. Awesome! You should be able to talk while you are exercising. After you are about 5 minutes into your workout, start to notice how easy it is to speak. At first, you may find that you can only say 2 to 3 words at a time. If you feel that you can carry on a conversation easily and say 5 to 6 words per breath, then you need to stop slacking. If you can't talk at all, then you need to reel it in. This method of judging how hard you are working is called the "talk test."

With that said, as you continue to work out on a regular basis, this threshold will change. Our bodies are super amazing in the fact that they adapt quickly. The more stress you apply to it through exercise, the more your body is going to be like "I got this. Now what!?!?!?" That's why I never tell my clients to get on a treadmill and run at a certain speed at a certain incline. Depending on what their body's physical abilities are will dictate how hard someone needs to be working. Factors like lack of sleep and stress can also play a part on how much your body can handle. Bottom line, notice how the words are coming out of your mouth every time you are breaking a sweat.

How Many Reps Does It Take to Get to the Center of a Good Workout?

There is so much confusion on how many reps to do and how to judge the right weight to use if doing something with resistance. For me, having correct form is the number 1 priority. Having been in the industry for a while, I can't tell you how many countless photos, Instagram videos, and just about anything on social media I have encountered where a fellow trainer is trying to impress others by pushing more weight than their body can handle. I'm not trying to be judgmental because I can't lift as much as them or that my muscles are not as big as theirs. My concern comes with sacrificing the integrity of the lumbar spine by trying to bench a ridiculous amount of weight or doing a barbell back squat with a weightlifting belt. It's my professional opinion that if you need the belt to support the trunk of your body then maybe it's just too heavy. I was 130 pounds and deadlifting a total of 225 pounds. Sans belt. Form is everything if you want your body to keep going for many years to come.

In the spotlight of wanting to lose weight, you will want to focus on a higher rep count of 15 to 20. The people training in the gym doing 1 to 3 reps are not training for the same purpose. Or if they are, they are likely misguided. As stated above, this isn't about some sloppy form while you flop all over the place. You want to make sure that your core is engaged (more on that later) and that you start with a neutral spine. Using a mirror to watch your form will at first help to improve your body awareness. To select the proper resistance for this rep range, you should feel that the last few reps are quite challenging. It doesn't matter if you are using weights or not. There are ways to manipulate your body to make things more challenging or if you need to tone it down a notch.

Core Tight!

This is definitely something that I remind my clients of on a regular basis. It is so easy to forget about those kazillion core muscles when you are trying to lunge here and press that. I get it. However, this is not a race. As you get used to moving your body in a multitude of ways, the less brainpower it will require, and you won't have to move super slow. I do think there is something to be said for moving with intention and awareness. When I am exercising, I like to think about the muscles I am using and really squeeze them on each contraction. Give them a friendly little "Hello!" It's time to work! Don't just go through the motions. Feel your entire body come together to complete each and every motion.

~~~~~*Core to Core*~~~~~

Activity 1:

If you aren't sure where your core is, try the following. Grab a trusted friend. You definitely wouldn't want to do this with someone you have pissed off recently or ever for that matter. With your hands behind your back, ask your good friend to act like they are going to punch you in the stomach but stopping around 6 inches away. Now that trust thing is making sense, huh? Even though you know they won't actually hit you, notice how your stomach tightens up as you brace for impact. This feeling may be the same you get when you step into a cold pool. Say hello to your core.

How did your body react? Did you feel the natural reaction of your spine to straighten? What other changes did you notice in your body?

Activity 2:

This activity can be done without having a partner ready to punch you in the stomach. Lay on the ground with your knees bent and feet flat on the floor. You will notice a natural curvature of your lumbar spine, which is also known as your lower back. Now actively press your lower back down into the mat so that your entire spine is close to being flat on the ground. When you do this, notice how your pelvis tilts towards the ground.

Does your belly tighten up like in the previous exercise? Do you find it hard to hold this position for longer than 10 to 15 seconds? If so, you can continue to practice these pelvic tilts to help strengthen the foundational muscles of your core. Working on this daily should allow you to see a vast improvement over a short period of time.

At first, it will be easier to just reflect back on these experiences when you need to engage your core. Over time, it will become second nature. Become familiar with what it is like to activate these muscle groups. As you continue to build on your fitness, this will always be your foundation.

~~~~~~~

Abs vs. Core—Below the Six-Pack

If I had a nickel for every time someone told me that they wanted to strengthen their core and then proceeded to show me a photo of defined abs in a magazine, then I would be a freaking billionaire living on my own tropical island with someone feeding me grapes. Look, abs and core are not the same things. Not even close. Your abdominal muscles that you know as a six-pack are known to us anatomy nerds as the rectus abdominis.

Your core muscles, on the other hand, are comprised of the following:
- •. Diaphragm
- •. Pelvic floor
- •. Internal obliques
- •. External obliques
- •. Transverse abdominis
- •. Multifidus
- •. Erector spinae
- •. Longissimus thoracis

Many of these muscles lie deep within your body to help support your spine and guide movement in the multiple directions that it can make. Side to side when you pick up luggage from the ground. In flexion when you set a box on the floor in front of you. From back to front such as when you are sitting up to get out of bed. You may not see the muscles like the cheese grater on some super hot 20 something male model, but they help you to do very basic functions on a regular basis. Strengthen your core, and you will reduce your chances of low back pain and hip discomfort as you age.

One of the most effective exercises to strengthen your core muscles is the plank. Achieving proper alignment for a plank is not hard, but I have definitely seen my fair share of planks that aren't doing crap for your core.

The setup can be done on your toes or with your knees on the ground and thigh bones at a slant:
- •. Think of setting up your body in a push-up position.
- •. Spread your fingers wide with your index finger pointing forward.
- •. Draw the crease of your elbow forward by rotating your upper-arm bone outward.
- •. Press your hands into the mat so that you round your shoulders down and pull your shoulder blades apart. This will round into your upper back.
- •. Pull your ribs in so that your belly is not dropping down to the ground. There should be no excessive arch in the low back.
- •. Tighten your quads by thinking of pulling your kneecaps up.
- •. Lift your hamstrings up.
- •. If doing this on your toes, see if you can lift high on to the balls of your feet.
- •. Your entire body should feel engaged. Remember to breathe!

You will want to work your way up to holding a plank for 1 to 2 minutes on your toes. If you are starting off on your knees, keep practicing until you can hold for 1 minute and then start practicing on your toes.

Do you have wrist issues? Do this on your forearms. You obviously won't be pressing your hands into the ground, but you can still rotate the upper-arm bones outward and press into your upper back. I don't believe in working through pain, but I definitely believe in finding a way to work around it. Otherwise, we would all just be full of lame excuses.

~~~~~ Test Time! ~~~~~

Now that you have practiced your form, it is time to see how long you can hold it. I don't care if it is 5 seconds on your knees. You need to know your truth. The cool thing will be when you notice yourself getting stronger and you can reflect back on this starting point. Need a distraction as you plank it? Put on a fun song that makes you want to go out and party on a Saturday night. My go-to is typically anything from Gwen Stefani, such as "Hollaback Girl." That song just gets me pumped and takes my mind off of what I am actually doing.

You totally got this! Use a timer to see how long you can hold your plank. Make whatever modifications you need to (use your knees or forearms) and notate. Try 3 times with 1 or 2 minutes of rest between.

1. _____

2. _____

3. _____

So how did you do? It was hard, I'm sure. You will get stronger over time the more you practice. Maybe even have a "plank off" next time you are with your workout buddy. See who can hold their plank the longest at the end of your workout. A little friendly competition never hurt anyone.

~~~~~~~

Fancy Equipment? Pieces You Have Around Your House!

This book is about not having the money to spend on fancy gym equipment or a studio membership. The good news is that you probably have items around your house that you can use, so you don't have to spend any money. All of the exercises in this book will not require you to have any equipment because you may need to spend it on other things, such as supporting your family or your business. The nice thing is that you really don't need fancy equipment to get into shape.

- •. **Furniture sliders**—There are fancy fitness gliders that you can use or you can use furniture sliders intended to move your couch for a fraction of the cost. Need something cheaper? You can use paper plates on a carpeted surface or socks on a hard surface, such as tile or hardwood. These are a great way to increase the core intensity of almost any exercise that has your hands or feet on the move.
- •. **Chairs or benches**—These serve as a great substitute for a weightlifting bench or plyo box. Of course, you will want to make sure that the furniture is steady and secure. If there is any wobble to it, I wouldn't recommend using it in your workout routine. Use common sense so you aren't put out of commission right from the start.
- •. **Plastic gallon jugs**—I am typically not a proponent for any drink that is sold in this type of container unless it is water; however, once such a container is empty, you can refill it with water to use as handheld weights. The exercises in this program will not require you to have these, but an up-level option will be given if that is appropriate for your fitness level.
- •. **Canned goods**—Grab those cans of garbanzo beans and do some bicep curls or shoulder presses. Small canned goods are great for challenging your upper body strength without having to buy expensive dumbbells.

Excuses That Fail

You've scheduled your workouts on your calendar, and you've set your goals. With this new sense of motivation, you will go far. That is until something gets in your way. It will happen, I promise. Even as a personal trainer, I battle excuses on a daily basis. I know that exercise is good for me (duh!), but it is hard for me to motivate sometimes too because I'm not a robot. I'm a human being with real struggles just like you. Having lived it and having helped my clients on a regular basis with these same struggles, I know you will be able to overcome them. It's all about being prepared to deal with these stupid little complications.

Top 5 Reasons to Skip Your Workout:

1. I Forgot My Gym Clothes!

As sexy as it may be to hit up the treadmill in heels, it is probably not safe or realistic. Make it easy to remember by packing your gym bag the night before and set it right in front of your door. Not next to it. Right in front of it so you would physically have to pick it up and move it to go to work.

2. I'm Starving!

It is not a good idea to work out on an empty stomach. If you haven't had a meal within a few hours, you will want to get some carbs in your body before working out. Unless you like getting dizzy, nauseous, and or just passing out all together. No bueno! Pack snacks regularly so you always have something, such as trail mix, an apple with peanut butter, or rollups (see snacks section in "What We Eat").

3. I'm Just Too Busy Today!

We're all busy. That's one of the reasons why you picked up this book because you don't have any time. Except you just did an activity where you found time in your schedule, right? It's easy to fill your time with surfing social media, binge-watching shows, or whatever. This is all about sprinkling it in any way you can. Why not binge-watch while you work out? I see no problem with it as long as you are getting your workout done. Be mindful of your time. Doing an exercise and then sitting down to watch your show for 10 minutes is not ok. You get the idea.

4. My Workout Buddy Cancelled!

This doesn't mean you have to scrap it all together. If it was a day that you were really looking forward to getting your sweat on, then go ahead and kill that workout. Maybe even take a post-workout sweaty pic and post it on social media. You will realize that you have a lot of support that extends beyond just your workout buddy. You can even tag me on Instagram @fun2befit_ceo, and I will be sure to give you a bravo!

5. It Is So Boring!

Sometimes you would rather poke your eyeballs out than even think about doing a squat or doing cardio. I get it. Having a physically active lifestyle since I was a teenager, it can feel so monotonous sometimes to have to work out. Things that can get me excited are trying something new in class, catching up with a friend over a hike, or having a crazy dance party. Dance party? Yup! I put on some awesome music and just start dancing. Inspired by the show Grey's Anatomy, dancing will almost always put you in a good mood and possibly motivate you to work out. If not, just keep on dancing and count it as your cardio! Sprinkle it in where you can baby!

Things to Remember

- •. Schedule your workouts like you would an important appointment you could not miss.
- •. Find ways to move more: stand more; walk more; just keep moving!
- •. Balance is key! Too much of anything will give you overactive muscles and eventually lead to injury. Mix up your workouts and include recovery days to feel good in your body.
- •. You don't need fancy gym equipment to get fit. Your body weight alone can do a lot. There are also plenty of things around your house you can utilize to add variety to your home workouts.
- •. Your will to become more fit is stronger than your weak excuses. Believe it, and find solutions.
- •. You are worth it!

The Workout

Dip Your Toes: 10 Day Plan

Starting something new can be scary, so I have put together this simple plan that will give you just a tiny taste. You will learn the basics that include foundational movements to get you started with good habits. Correct form and working towards a full range of motion will give you the skills you need to be able to move towards variations of the fundamentals.

Remember, this is not about being perfect. You are learning, so start by having patience with yourself. We are not all athletically inclined and coordinated. We all do, however, have the same 24 hours in a day, and we all have the ability just to try.

Day 1
Squats
Lunges
Bridges
Donkey kicks
Side Lying Leg Lifts
Day 2
Smooth move day: walk, hike, yoga, bike

Day 3

Pushups

Back extension

Triceps dips

Plank

Single-leg Lifts

Day 4

Cardio: walk, hike, bike

Day 5

Side Lunges

Walkouts

Side Planks

Single-Leg Extensions

Shuffle Squats

Day 6

Smooth move day

Day 7

Rest: grocery shopping, meal prep for week, stretch

Day 8

Squats

Lunges

Bridges

Donkey Kicks

Side-Lying Leg Lifts

Day 9

Smooth move day

Day 10

Pushups

Back Extension

Triceps dips

Plank

Single-Leg Lifts

Take The Plunge - 28 Day Plan

Day 11
Cardio: walk, hike, bike
Day 12
Reverse Lunges

Plank Shoulder Taps

Russian Twists

Clam Shells

Alternating Froggers (on bench or chair)
Day 13
Smooth move day
Day 14
Rest: grocery shopping, meal prep for week, stretch
Day 15
Plie Squats

Crossover Lunges

Supermans

Quadruped Leg Lifts

Lying Adductor Leg Lifts
Day 16
Smooth move day: walk, hike, yoga, bike
Day 17
Kneeling Triceps Pushups

Pronated Y Raises

Side-Lying Triceps Pushups

Kickdowns

Plank Walks
Day 18
Cardio: walk, hike, bike
Day 19
Reverse Lunges

Plank Shoulder Taps

Russian Twists

Clam Shells

Alternating Froggers (on bench or chair)

Day 20

Smooth move day

Day 21

Rest: grocery shopping, meal prep for week, stretch

Day 22

Plie Squats

Crossover Lunges

Supermans

Quadruped leg lifts

Lying Adductor Leg Lifts

Day 23

Smooth move day: walk, hike, yoga, bike

Day 24

Kneeling Triceps Pushups

Pronated Y Raises

Side-Lying Triceps Pushups

Kickdowns

Plank Walks

Day 25

Cardio: walk, hike, bike

Day 26

Reverse Lunges

Plank Shoulder Taps

Russian Twists

Clam Shells

Alternating Froggers (on bench or chair)

Day 27

Smooth move day

Day 28

Congrats!!! You made it! Keep the momentum going.

Rest: grocery shopping, meal prep for week, stretch

The Exercises

Alternating Froggers

1. Start in a plank position with your shoulders directly over your wrists.
2. Step your right foot outside your right hand.
3. Return to plank position and perform on opposite side. That is 1 rep.

Make it harder: Instead of returning back to plank position, explosively jump your feet from the right side to left side so that you skip the plank.

Make it easier: Put your hands up higher on to a chair or couch.

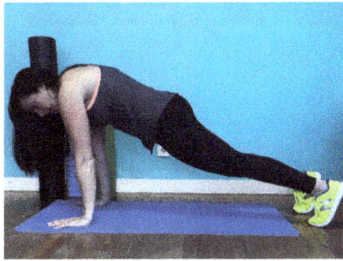

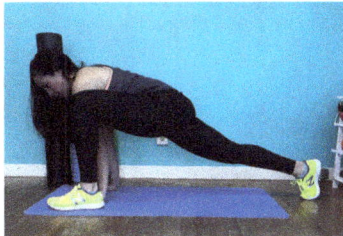

Back Extension

1. Lay on your stomach with your arms by your side and palms facing to the ground.
2. Lift your chest, arms, and legs up but keep your neck neutral by looking down, so you don't strain your neck.
3. Hold for 2 seconds and then return to the ground.

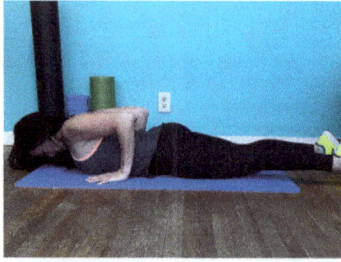

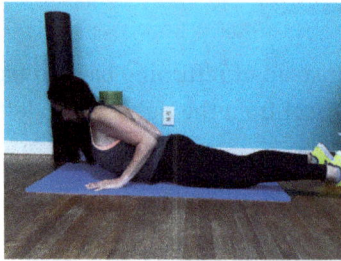

Bridges

1. Lay on your back with your knees bent and feet flat on the floor.
2. Press your hips up and your feet into the ground as you squeeze your booty and the back of your legs. Lower back down.

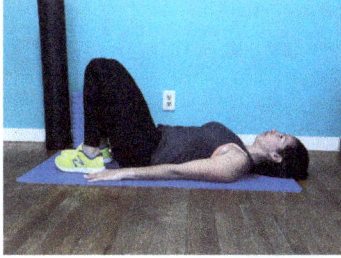

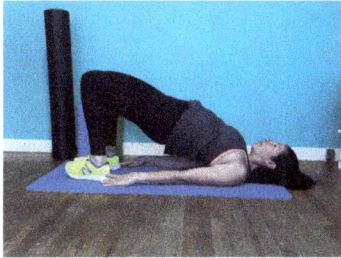

Clam Shells

1. Lay on your side with your knees bent at 90 degrees.
2. Bring your knees in front of you so that your feet and hips are lined up.
3. Keeping your feet together, separate your knees, and squeeze the outer glute muscle.
4. Lower your leg back down, bringing the knees back together.

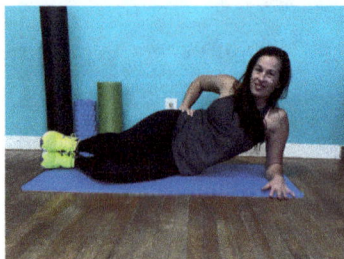

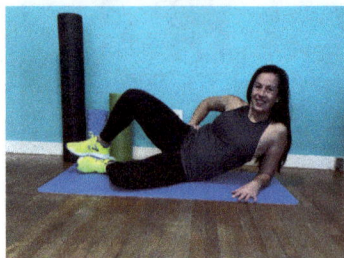

Crossover Lunges

1. Start by standing with your feet together.
2. With your right foot, take a big step backwards and behind and across the left leg.
3. Bend both knees to lower back down to the ground without actually touching your knees to the ground. Pressing in to the left foot, step your right foot back next to your left.
4. Repeat on the other side. That is 1 rep.

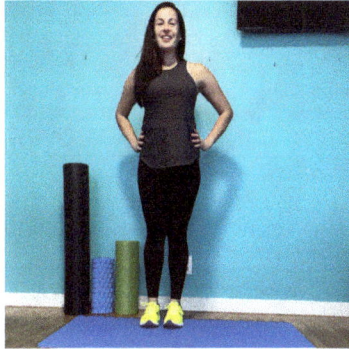

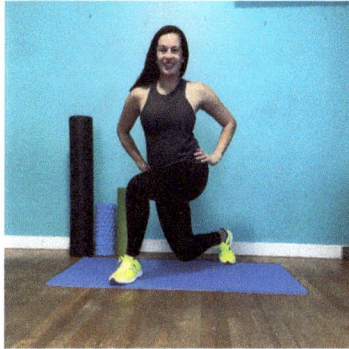

Donkey Kicks

1. Get into a kneeling position with the shoulders over the wrists and hips over the knees.
2. Flex both ankles so your toes are pointing to the ground.
3. Keeping your right knee bent, press your right foot up towards the ceiling and squeeze your right glute.
4. Lower your right knee down back to starting position.

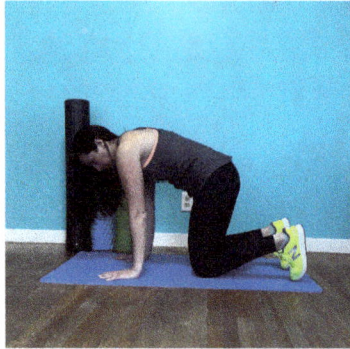

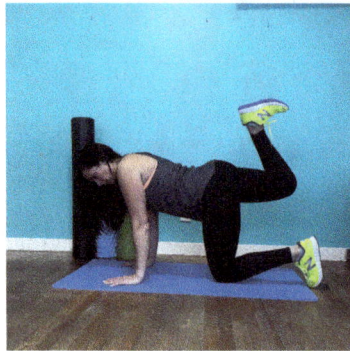

Kickdowns

1. Lay on your back with your legs straight in the air so your feet are directly over your hips.
2. Press your low spine down into the ground.
3. Keeping your entire spine flat on the surface, start to lower your legs to the ground.
4. Only lower your legs as low as you can while maintaining the integrity of the low back to the ground.
5. Lift the legs back up to starting position.

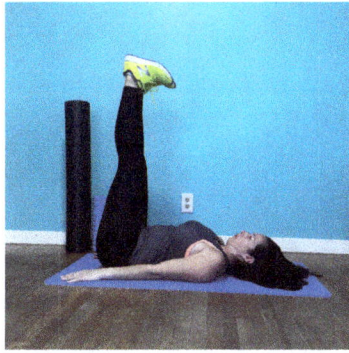

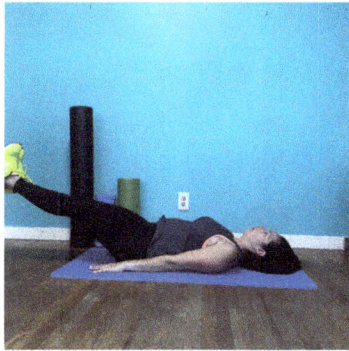

Kneeling Triceps Pushups

1. Start in a plank position, but with your knees on the ground.
2. Check that your shoulders are directly over your wrists.
3. Keeping your body completely straight, slowly lower yourself towards the ground, with the upper arms squeezing the sides of your body.
4. If your elbows flare out to the sides, you risk injuring your shoulders over time.
5. Press yourself back up to starting position.

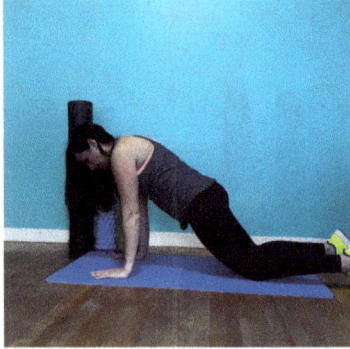

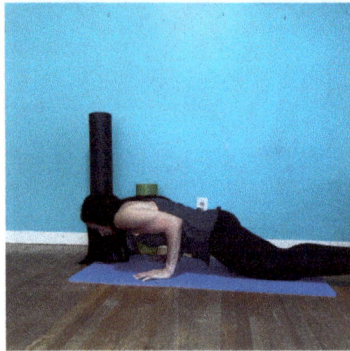

Lunges

1. Starting from standing with your feet together take a large step forward with your right foot.
2. Bending both knees, slowly lower yourself to the ground to hover your back knee.
3. Check that your knee and ankle are stacked in your front leg and your knee is under the hip of the back leg.
4. Press into the right heel to step the feet back to center.

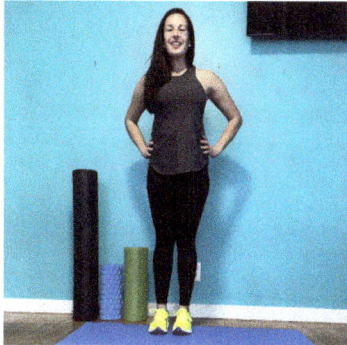

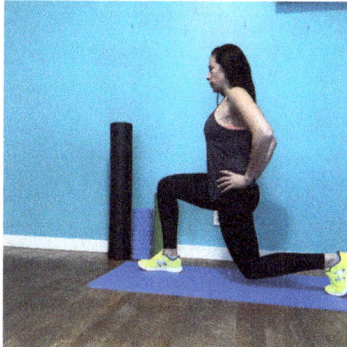

Plank

1. Get into a kneeling position with your shoulders directly over your wrists.
2. Extend 1 leg straight behind you with your toes on the ground.
3. Extend the other leg straight.
4. If this is too challenging, lower both knees down to the ground.
5. Keep the body straight so that the hips are in a straight line with your feet/knees and shoulders.

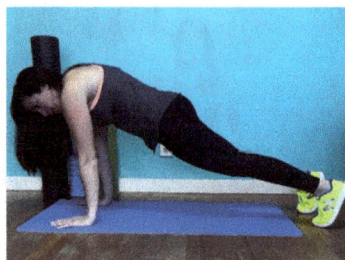

Plank Shoulder Taps

1. Form a plank position on your toes or knees.
2. Pick up your right hand and tap your left shoulder.
3. Place your right hand back down to starting position.
4. Repeat the same with your left hand. That is 1 rep.

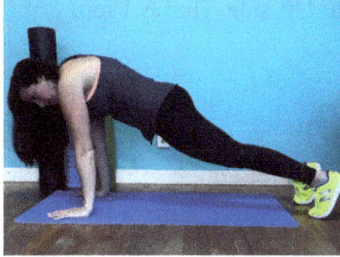

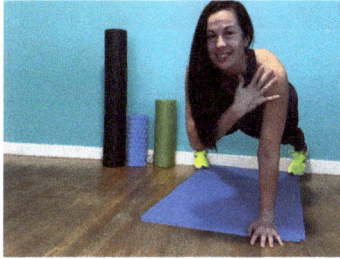

Plank walks

1. Start in a plank position from your toes or knees.
2. Lower on to your forearms while maintaining a straight body.
3. You are now in forearm plank!
4. Push up with your right hand back to the plank position on your hands.
5. Repeat on your left side. That is 1 rep.

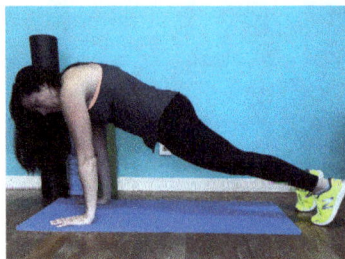

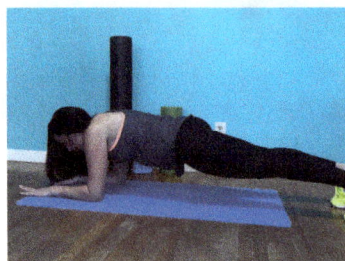

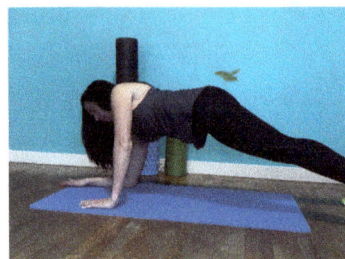

Plie Squats

1. From a standing position, take your feet out wider than your hips.
2. Turn your toes outward 45 degrees.
3. Leading with your hips, start to lower your body like you want to sit down onto a chair.
4. If you are new to doing squats, I would recommend practicing with a chair or bench under you.
5. Press into your heels and straighten your legs to come back up to a standing position.

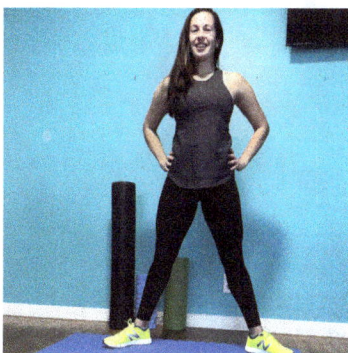

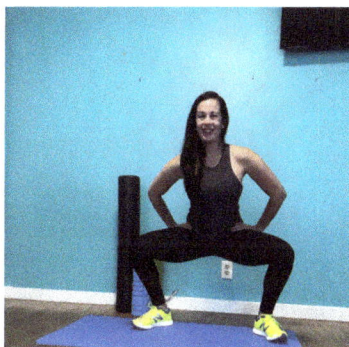

Pronated Y Raises

1. Lay down on your belly.
2. Reach your arms overhead with your thumbs up towards the ceiling.
3. Press the tops of your feet down into the ground.
4. Lift your chest and arms off the ground, squeezing your back muscles and butt.
5. Lower yourself back to the ground.

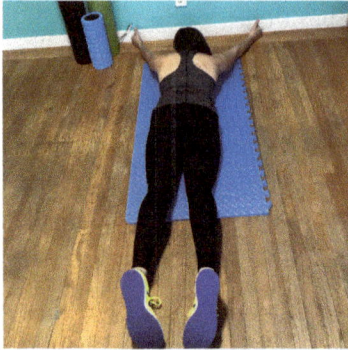

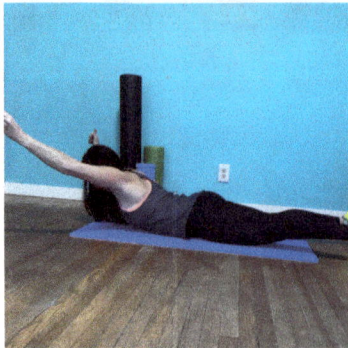

Pushups

1. Start in a plank position but with your hands slightly wider than your shoulders.
2. Lower your body in a straight line down to the ground, bending your elbows out and back.
3. Press evenly through your palms to come back up to your starting position.

Make it easier: Come into an inclined position by placing your hands on a bench, countertop, or the back of your couch. The incline position makes it easier for your upper body while still working your core.

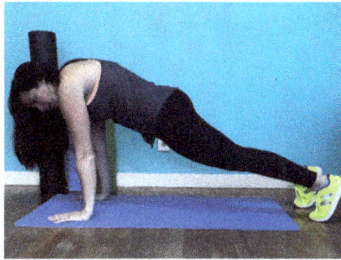

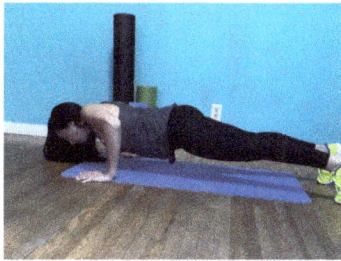

Quadruped Leg Lifts

1. Start in an all fours position.
2. Extend your right leg out to the side with your foot flexed so that your toes are pulling towards your shin.
3. Lift your right leg up as high as you can without leaning over to your left side.
4. Keep your left arm straight!
5. Lower your right leg back down to the ground.

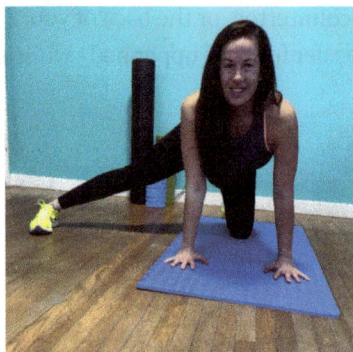

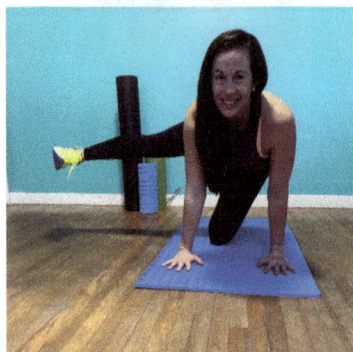

Reverse Lunges

1. From a standing position, take a large step back with the toes of your right foot on the ground.
2. Bend both of your knees, keeping the front knee stacked over the front ankle and the back knee under your hip.
3. Press in to your left heel and step forward to bring the feet back together.

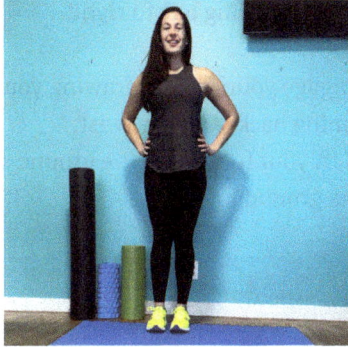

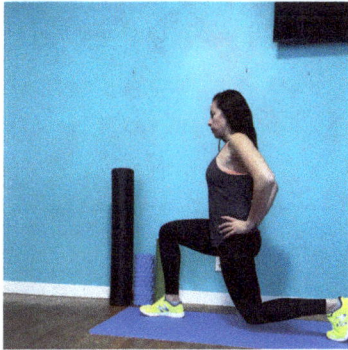

Russian Twists

1. Sit down on the ground with your knees bent and toes up.
2. Lean back just to the point where you feel your belly tighten up.
3. Avoid rounding the shoulders forward and pull them back to maintain a flat back.
4. Extend your arms straight in front of your and press your palms together.
5. Twist your arms, reaching left to right.

Make it easier: Engage your core by drawing your belly button inward, but avoid leaning back. Add the twist.

Make it harder: Lift your feet up off the ground so that your shins are parallel with the ground.

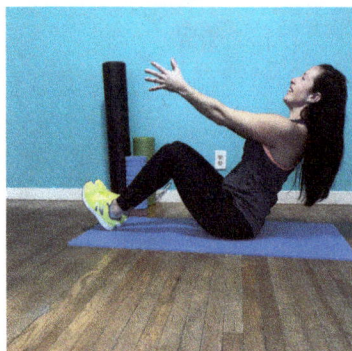

Shuffle Squats

1. Get into a squat position with your feet slightly wider than your hips.
2. Place your hands at your waist.
3. Lower down into your squat by leading with the hips.
4. Press through your heels to come up to standing and step your left foot to your right.
5. Step out with your right foot and squat back down.
6. Press through your heels to stand and step your right foot to your left.
7. Step out with your left and lower back down into your squat.
8. Continue to repeat stepping side to side.

Make it harder: Add more of an explosive movement by popping up from your squat so it is almost a jumping motion.

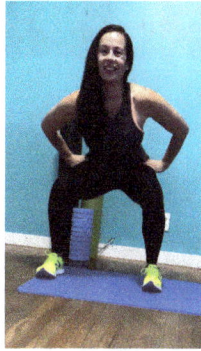

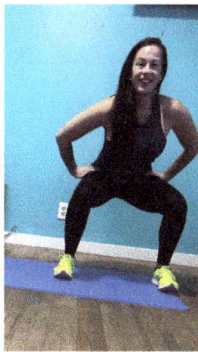

Side Lunges

1. Start from a standing position and step out to the side with your right foot.
2. Leading only with your hips, bend into your right knee as you keep your left leg straight.
3. Press off from your right foot and bring both feet back together.
4. Repeat on the left leg. That is 1 rep.

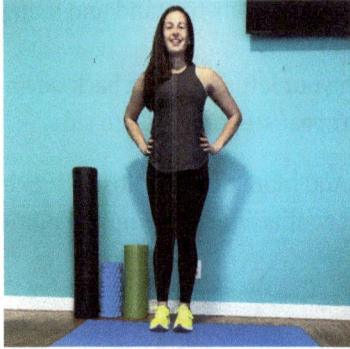

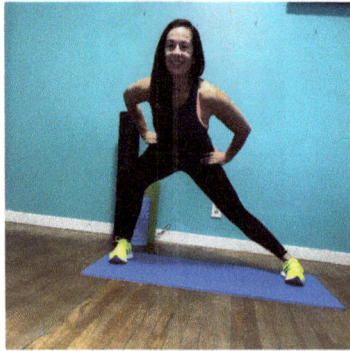

Side-Lying Abductor Leg Lifts

1. Lying on your left side with your legs straight, bring your right leg in front of you so your right hip is extended 90 degrees.
2. Flex your right ankle so that your toes are pulling towards your face, lift your right leg as high as you can.
3. Lower your right leg back down to the ground without touching and lift back up.

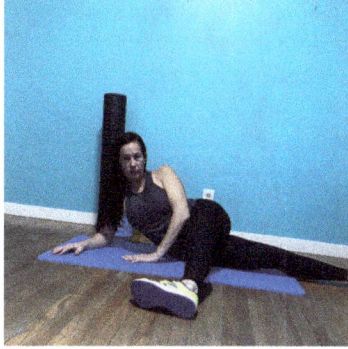

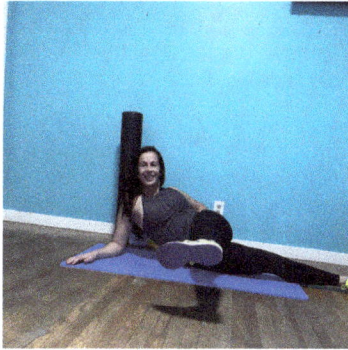

Side-Lying Adductor Leg Lifts

1. Laying on your right side with your legs straight, take your left foot and place it on the ground with a bent knee.
2. Your left foot will be behind your right leg on the ground.
3. Flex your right toes so they are pulling towards your face.
4. Lift your right leg up as high as you can.
5. Lower back down.

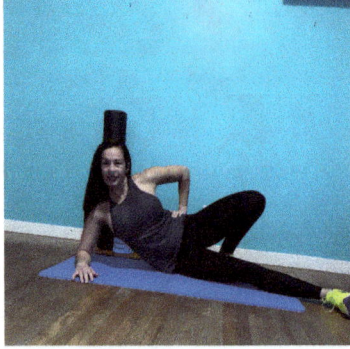

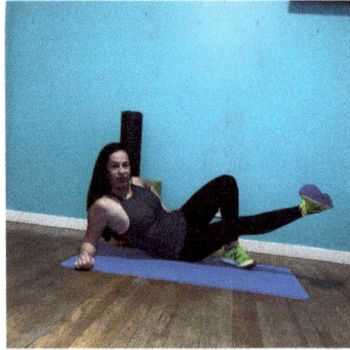

Side-Lying Triceps Pushup

1. Lie on your left side with your knees bent.
2. Take your left arm and wrap it around your belly like you are hugging yourself.
3. Place your right hand in front of your left shoulder.
4. Pressing into your right hand, straighten your right arm completely to lift your upper body up off the ground.
5. Lower yourself back down slowly.

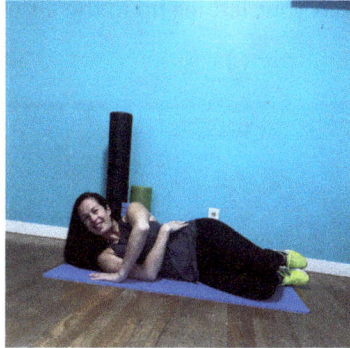

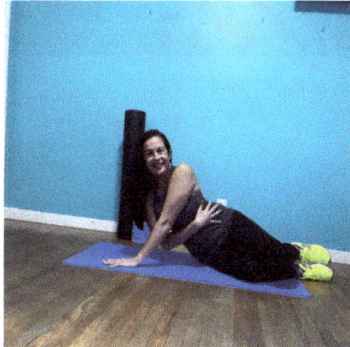

Side Plank

1. Lying on your right side, prop yourself up with your right hand.
2. With your legs straight, lift your hips up off the ground so that your body is in a straight line.
3. You can rest your left arm by your side or reach it straight up in the air.

Make it easier: Lower your right knee down to the ground for extra support.

Make it harder: Lift your left leg up in the air to hover over your right.

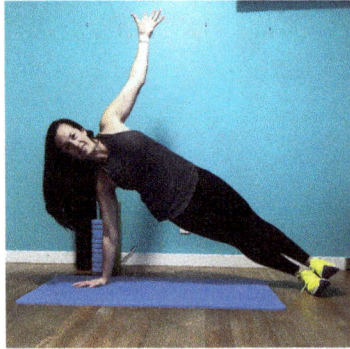

Single Leg Lifts

1. Lying on your back, take both feet in the air with your legs straight.
2. Flex your feet by pulling your toes down towards your face.
3. Press your lower back down into the ground to achieve a flat spine.
4. Maintaining a flat back, lower your right leg down to the ground as low as you can.
5. Lift your leg back up and repeat with the left leg. That is 1 rep.

Make it easier: Just don't drop your leg that low to the ground.
Make it harder: Lower both legs at the same time.

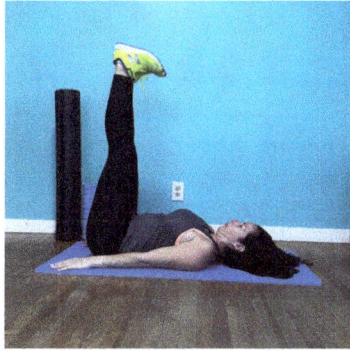

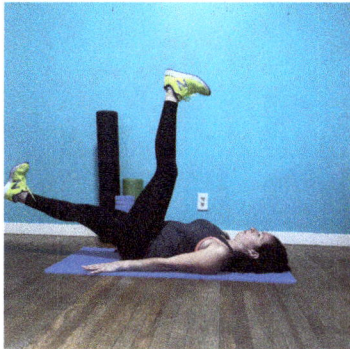

Single Leg Extensions

1. Lying on your back, bring your legs into a table-top position with your feet lifted and your knees directly over your hips.
2. Press the lower spine down into the ground.
3. Keeping this connection, extend your right leg out straight and towards the ground while maintaining the spinal connection.
4. Pull your right knee back into the starting position.
5. Repeat the same with your left leg. That is 1 rep.

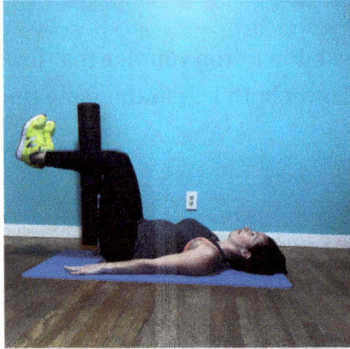

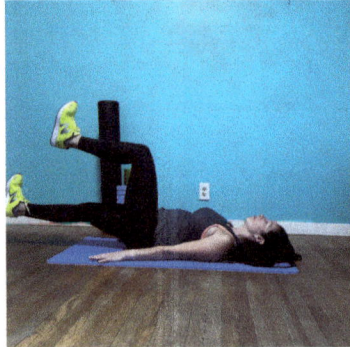

Superman

1. Lie on your belly.
2. Reach your arms overhead with your palms facing down on the ground.
3. Lift your arms, legs, and chest while keeping your eyes looking down.
4. Lower yourself back down to the ground.

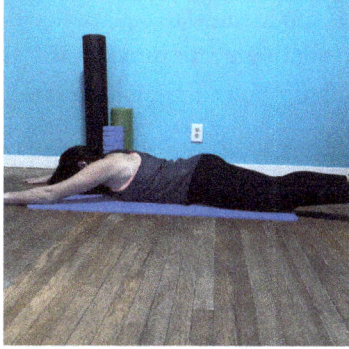

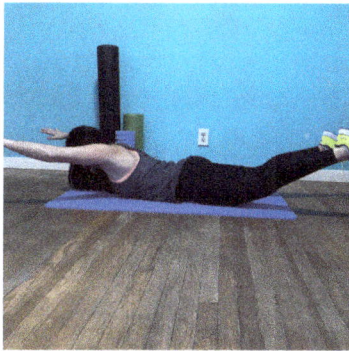

Squats

1. From a standing position, take your feet slightly wider than your hips.
2. Leading with your hips, start to lower down as if you were sitting in a chair.
3. Press through your heels to come back up to the standing position.

Make it easier: If you are new to squats, you can place a chair or bench underneath you. Aim your hips towards the seat under you. If you lose your balance, you can simply sit down.

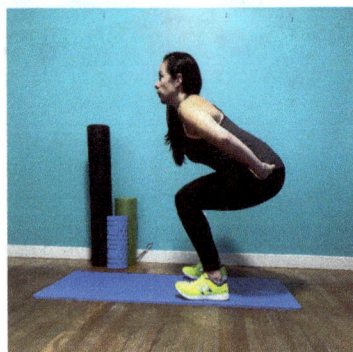

Triceps Dip

1. Using a bench or chair, sit down on the edge.
2. Place your hands on whatever you are sitting on with your fingers pointing towards your butt and slightly wider than your hips.
3. Lift your butt up and shift forward so you are directly in front of the edge.
4. Bend your elbows to lower yourself down.
5. Make sure that your elbows point behind you and not out to the side.
6. Press through the heel of your hand to bring yourself back up.

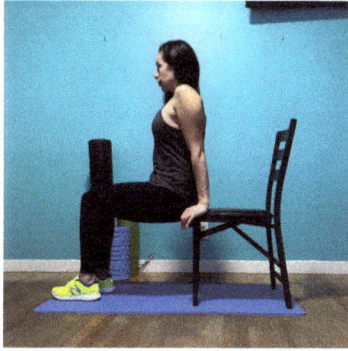

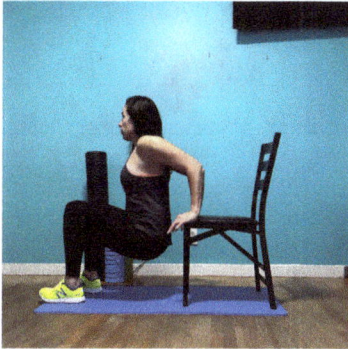

Walkouts

1. From a standing position, place your hands down on the ground by bending from the waist and also bending your knees as much as needed.
2. Walk your hands out until you've reached a plank position.
3. Walk your hands back to your feet, bending your knees as much as needed.
4. Bring yourself back up to a standing position by drawing your belly in.

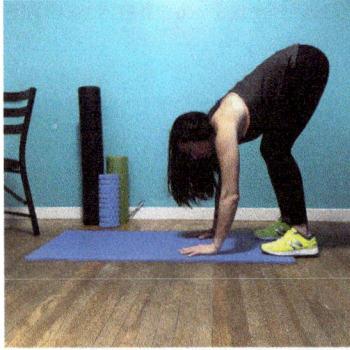

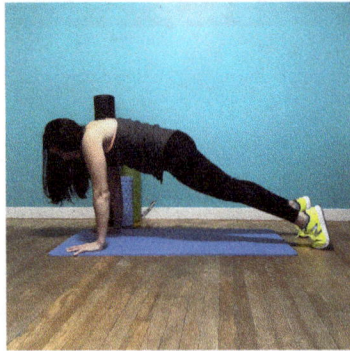

Part 4:

Finding Balance

Nutrition and exercise are definitely a huge factor in living healthy in your body. If you have these two things down, you are likely to feel good in your skin. Want to feel even better? There are other

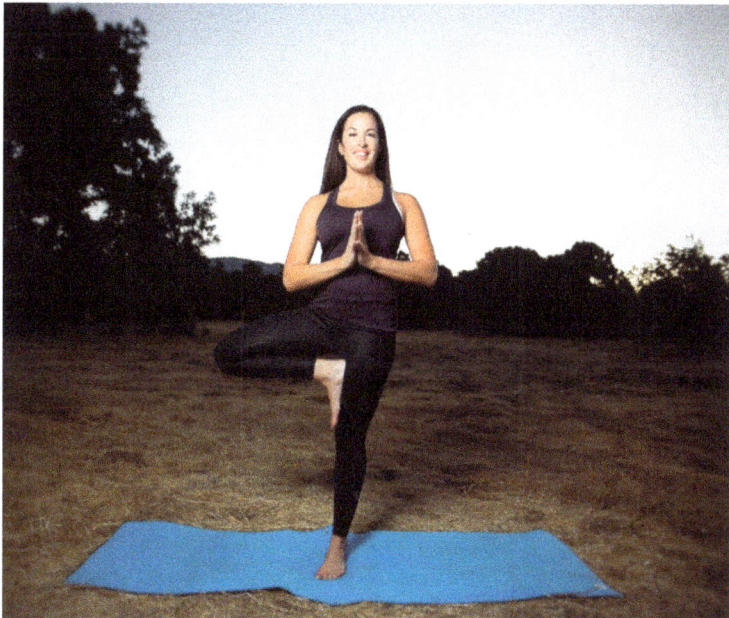

teeny tiny tweaks you can make that will help you to make healthier food choices and tackle that workout with a bit more vigor. Don't make this new lifestyle change harder than it needs to be. Discover ways that you can completely take control of your life and hold on hard to this new you!

All about Sleep

Get Your Zzzzz's

I will be the first to tell you that sometimes it is difficult to get a good night's sleep. How do you think this book got done while I was working as a full-time personal trainer? The amount of good sleep varies from person to person, but typically 7 to 8 hours a night ensures proper recovery. Ever notice how good you feel when you get a good night's rest? Your energy is up. You can think clearly. You can make easier healthy food choices. You're ready to have an awesome workout.

Now think about those nights that you got less than 6 hours of sleep. For my friends out there who are parents that get only 2 to 3 consecutive hours, I give a hat off to you. You know what it feels like to have a complete and utter lack of sleep, leaving you feeling like you want to curl up in a ball and hide from the world. Maybe it's not that extreme, but a lack of sleep has likely made it easier to say yes to junk food and no to that workout.

I don't want to bore you too much with the science. However, there are some major advantages to getting your snooze on. It is recommended that 7 to 8 hours of sleep is an ideal amount for adults. According to Shalini Paruthi, MD, a sleep specialist and spokesperson for the American Academy of Sleep Medicine, these are the top 5 health benefits of sleep:

#1: Healthy Heart

According to Dr. Paruthi, a lack of sleep is linked directly to a whole slew of heart problems, including high blood pressure and heart disease. Cortisol also comes into play, which is altered by levels of stress and is linked to belly fat (more on that in a moment). Since cortisol is directly connected to stress in the body, it sends messages to your heart to work harder. When you rest, your heart also rests. End of story.

#2: Weight Management

As mentioned in #1, the stress hormone cortisol is linked to an increase in belly fat. Here's how: When your body releases extra cortisol, it triggers your body to then release the hunger hormone known as ghrelin. On the flip side, it decreases the production of leptin, a hormone which is responsible for telling your brain when you are full. You can probably see where this is going, right? You have more hormones telling you that you need to eat and fewer hormones telling you that you are full, which leads to you eating more. The cherry on the top is that people that are hungry due to lack of sleep tend to crave foods that are both high in calories and fat. These cravings are real, and I get it. Manage your hormones better by stopping the binge-watching and going to bed.

#3: Fewer Accidents

Recall the horrible destruction of the space shuttle Challenger and the massive oil spill of the Exxon Valdez? These were both attributed to sleep deprivation. I personally was pushing myself so hard for a short time with my health and wellness business under minimal sleep, and I got into 2 car accidents in 2 weeks. These were my first accidents ever in 22 years! According to the National Academy of Medicine, 1 in 5 auto accidents in the United States is due to "drowsy driving." That's approximately 1 million crashes per year. Be safe ... don't sleep and drive.

#4: Immune System

Sick and tired of being sick and tired? Getting ample amounts of rest helps to keep the cells and proteins of your immune system better able to ward off that pesky cold, flu, or other illness. There are also foods that you can consume that are high in antioxidants (think greens and berries) that when combined with regular, good sleep can keep you from feeling hit by a sledgehammer and in tip-top shape.

#5: Foggy Brain

Ever go through your day feeling in a daze and not quite able to focus? A lack of sleep is kind of like that childhood game where you put your forehead on a bat and spin around multiple times and then try to walk. You are disoriented, confused, and likely to make a mistake that you normally wouldn't. Just one poor night of sleep can spill over into your day. This has the possibility of affecting your performance at work by causing you to make mistakes. The bad part is that you may not even realize that you made a mistake. Not exactly how you want to get ahead in your job.

Recapture Your Zzzzz's

So you get it. You need to sleep, but how? Maybe you have a hard time falling asleep, or maybe you need to reprioritize your responsibilities so you hit the sack at a reasonable hour. Regardless of why you haven't been sleeping enough, here are some of my habits that I find help to aid me in my sleeping process.

Power Off

Living in Silicon Valley, it seems that everything is electronic-based. Just look at how much we rely on our cell phones these days and the capability to stream our favorite shows. There has been a multitude of studies that show the benefits of stepping away from your TV, cell phone, tablet, laptop, and anything else electronic at least 1 hour before bed. It gives your brain the opportunity to disconnect and decrease the amount of stimulation so that you can start to unwind completely.

Essential Oils

Ever walk into a spa to get a massage and notice how you instantly feel relaxed by the scents in the air? I know I do! My favorite scent to calm my mind is eucalyptus. You can find many essential oils on Amazon, either sold solo or in kits. Not only do I like putting these into my diffuser at night before bed, but I also keep a bottle in my car to calm my nerves while commuting in traffic. While you can't get rid of all of the idiot drivers out on the road, you can help regulate how you react to them and all of the other b.s. that happens every day. Try putting a couple of drops between your palms and rubbing them together. Then place them in front of your face and take a few deep breaths. Creating this calming environment with a diffuser sets the mood to melt off the tension from your day and let you snuggle under those sheets for a good night's sleep.

Bubble Bath

You don't necessarily need the bubbles, but you could use bath salts or your favorite good smelling bodywash. Or maybe even add in that essential oil you love. My baths are a ritual with candles, a glass of red wine, and some relaxing tunes. The warm water will help to release tension in your muscles, and just laying there for a moment will feel like a much-needed break in your day. Sometimes, I even put on a face mask, so I truly bring the spa home to me.

Self-Massage

This is something that I don't do enough, but every time I do, I can't figure out why I don't make more time for it. It would be wonderful if we could have the time and money to go to the spa multiple times per week. The reality is that most of us don't. There are numerous self-massage tools available out there. Some of my favorites to use are foam rollers (choose something soft if you are really stiff) and Yoga Tune Up balls. The balls are great because they are tiny enough to fit into any gym bag or purse. They can also fit into almost any little nook and cranny of your body. Need a little neck rub? These guys will do the trick. I will discuss later how this is an integral part of functional movement for long-term mobility.

Meditation

Sitting in one spot for a period of time is definitely not something that comes easily to me. I seriously would be super antsy and fidgety. However, using one of the meditation apps that I have downloaded on my phone makes it easier to shut my mind off for 5 to 10 minutes. Meditation takes practice, so don't get frustrated if after a few minutes you can't sit still. My favorite app to use is Calm, and I occasionally switch it up with Headspace. Both are free! You can also simply just sit in a relaxing atmosphere, close your eyes, and breathe. Keep reading to learn some very simple breathing techniques I use for myself as well as when I am teaching yoga classes.

The Melting Zone

Did you just have that day, or maybe even a week, from hell? Implement all 4 of these techniques for one banging tension melter. Rub a couple of drops of essential oil between your palms and breathe it in while you run your bath water. Add more oil to your water or some bath salts while you sip on a glass of wine or tea. Now that your muscles are relaxed, you can massage out any kinks you have with your fave self-massage tool. To top it off, take 5 to 10 minutes to meditate. Head to bed, and melt away without a care in the world.

Don't Be a Cactus; Be a Fish

A cactus is easy for me to take care of because I am absolutely horrible at remembering to water my plants. Matter of fact, I don't buy any plants that need to be watered regularly because it just won't happen. On the opposing end, you have a fish. Fish always stay hydrated and are constantly surrounded by water. Be a fish! Some people are really good about drinking water. If I don't carry water with me, I honestly won't drink it.

Know that what you get hydrated by doesn't have to be just plain water. The only time I want to drink plain water is when I am working out. On a day to day basis, I like to enjoy sparkling infused waters or flat infused waters (inspiration from my recipes posted in Part 2). Unsweetened tea is another great option. To make sure that you consume enough H2O on a daily basis, take your body weight in pounds and divide that by 2 and voilà! If you weigh 140 pounds, then 70 ounces of water should be your target. That's how much you want to aim for to moisten your lips. When you work out, you are losing water through sweat, so make sure you make up for that. About 8 to 10 ounces should get you rehydrated for every 30 to 40 minutes of strenuous exercise. Remember, a fish, not a cactus.

Smart Like Doogie Howser, MD

I may be dating myself by referencing the Doogie, but if you are unfamiliar with the TV show, it was based on a teenage prodigy that was a doctor. Your muscles are surprisingly just as smart. If you have ever in your life started a workout program, you will remember how sore you were after that first session. As you continued on with your "routine," it became easier as your muscles got stronger and the soreness went away. Creating variability in exercise will keep your body guessing so it never adapts to the same old routine. You will achieve an afterburn effect by breaking down muscle to create microtears that require the muscle to repair itself which translate to being sore. This basically means that you are burning calories after your workout. Hell yeah!

The thing is that your muscles are super-adaptable. Muscles develop a memory of movement, which also includes load bearing and endurance. I see so many people hit a wall and plateau, and they can't seem to figure out why they stop seeing changes. The truth is that if you don't switch up what you are doing every couple of weeks, your muscles will get used to the movements. This book gives you the basics of foundational types of exercises. Once you get these down, you can add weight, increase the reps, and change the direction or range of motion to continue adding stress to your body for continued change. Consistency and variation will be the key to seeing results and improving strength.

Chill Out and Recover

Finally! Time to relax. This getting fit stuff is hard work. I agree; it can really be exhausting and trust me, your body is also craving a bit of rest. There are so many ways that you can take advantage of your rest day, and recovery is just as important as the exercise and nutrition aspect.

Here are my favorite ways to relax, but feel free to add on anything that is fun for you:
- •. Hiking with a friend: This is such a great way to catch up on life and get some extra steps in your day.
- •. Water sports: If you live near a body of water, you can go kayaking, paddleboating, and stand-up paddleboarding. Just remember to wear your sunscreen!
- •. Self-care: This could be doing a Yoga Tune Up sequence on your neck and shoulders to relieve stress from your week. Or maybe doing some gentle yoga stretches from one of the sequences in this book.
- •. Walking everywhere: Depending on where you live, take advantage of errands that are walkable, or maybe head to your local farmer's market. I am in a rush most days, but when I'm not, I like walking to get a pedicure or a massage or picking up a few things from the grocery store.
- •. Biking: Where I live, we have tons of bike-friendly streets and trails. Maybe you can take your kids with you and turn it into some family time as well.

Inhale the Good Stuff

No, I am not suggesting that you resort to drugs to calm down and de-stress. Taking time just to breathe is such a simple way to calm your mind, yet many of us don't. Putting yourself in an environment free of distractions (this may be for a few minutes in your car after sitting in traffic to get to work) by closing your eyes and focusing on your breath is a great way for you to refocus and calm the sympathetic nervous system. If you can have a clear mind, you will feel less stressed, frustrated, and you will be able to think with clarity.

Benefits of decreasing activation of your sympathetic nervous system:
- •. Decrease of stress hormones
- •. Lower blood pressure
- •. Better sleep quality
- •. Less muscle tension
- •. Reduced anxiety
- •. Improved function of the immune and digestive systems

All of this sounds great, but if it is all about breathing, aren't we all already doing that? I mean, you know how to breathe right? Obviously, or you wouldn't be reading this book right now if you weren't. The question is, how do you control your breathing so that you can reap the benefits of meditation and feel like you are in charge of your life?

~~~~~Breath Awareness~~~~

Time to put this into practice. Find a comfortable place that is free of distractions. Again, this can literally be anywhere: sitting in a parked car with the radio off; lying down in bed with your knees bent to support the lower back; getting comfortable on a pillow on the floor. You can set a timer for a few minutes if you like or just decide to enjoy for as long as it is restful. If you do set a timer, I would suggest something that is easy on the ears, such as chimes or a piano and less similar to a car alarm. You don't want your heart to skip a beat and jolt you out of this state of calm. Once you feel comfortable, go ahead and close your eyes.

The following is a guide to breath awareness. You can record yourself saying these lines slowly, have someone read it to you, or just read it to yourself before putting it into practice.

"Start to notice your breath as it moves in and out of your body. Bring awareness to how long each inhale and exhale is. See if you can start to expand them and make each inhale and exhale a little bit longer. Take notice of the small pause between each breath. Enjoy this moment. Do you feel any areas of tension in your body? See if you can start to relax those spots with every exhale you take. Feel how your chest and belly stretch with every inhale. Allow your shoulders to relax as your belly and chest deflate on every exhale. Keep your jaw loose so there is a little bit of space between your teeth. Stay here in this relaxed state for as long as you like."

~~~~~Breath Count~~~~~

Another simple way to calm your mind and body down is with breath count. It has a similar effect as counting to 10 when you are feeling super pissed off at someone or something. Begin by finding a comfortable position and a place free of distraction. Place your right hand on your belly and your left hand over your heart. Close your eyes.

On your next inhale count 1, 2, 3. Hold your breath for 1, 2, 3. Exhale 1, 2, 3. Hold 1, 2, 3. Continue this count on your own. As you count, feel the ebb and flow of your breath. Notice the rise and fall of your belly and chest as your hands float up and as they slowly descend closer to you. Continue with this count for as long as you feel comfortable.

~~~~~ Creating Your Oasis ~~~~~

To me, an oasis is this cool, dreamy place that makes me feel close to being on vacation. Unless you are retired with endless amounts of money, you likely can't just go anywhere at the drop of a dime. However, you can create an inviting space in your home that will be perfect for your meditations and yoga stretches (see the upcoming sequences). After all, the thought of going on vacation just sounds so relaxing, doesn't it? This oasis will help you set the tone and be the happy place you can always turn to.

To set up, you will want to find a space in your home that you can use. This can be a corner of your living room or office. You really don't need a lot of space. The next thing you will need is something that you can put stuff on, such as a small table, chair, stool, or bookshelf. Now for the fun part! You will want to choose things that make you feel happy and calm. I like to include different elements that stimulate my senses.

Items you may want to include:
- •. Candles or incense that creates a glow as well as a pleasant scent.
- •. Plants that offer color and help to purify the air.
- •. Maybe a water feature that emits a peaceful sound.
- •. You could also have photos of loved ones or places that you love to visit.

There is no right or wrong to this. Different things make different people happy. Choose the things that you like so that you will be encouraged to take some time for yourself to relax and feel human again.

Flexibility vs. Stability: What's the Difference?

The words "flexibility" and "stability" sound almost the same, but you can have one without the other. Most people understand what being flexible means. A lot of us were more flexible when we were younger, and somehow it dissipated into thin air as we grew older. Here we are as adults walking around all stiff and unable to touch our toes. To feel better in your bodies, there are a few things to consider. Now that you have started exercising, have you taken the time to stretch after? Do you have any areas that always seem to remain tight, no matter what the exercise? If you get a massage, do you still retain knots? If you are flexible, do you notice that you seem to be weak around certain joints?

Not all of these questions may make sense, but we will dive into all of it. The true definition of flexibility according to Wikipedia is range of movement in a joint or series of joints, and length in muscles that cross the joints to induce a bending movement or motion. Flexibility sounds like a good thing right? The problem is, that the joints need strength as much pliability. A lack of stabilization can cause major issues to muscles and joints such as tears, strains, and joint deterioration. Ouch!

Finding stability within your joints allows this junction of bone to move with control and at times hold a position with the assistance of supporting joints. If the muscles are inflexible, the joint can't move as freely as it is intended to. On the other hand, when you have

152 • RESHAPE YOUR HEALTH

a lack of strength, your joints are at risk for going beyond their limits and potentially creating an injury. Both flexibilty and stability are important for your body. They go together like peanut butter and jelly.

Bend So
You Don't Break

We all know we should be doing more of it, but do we really make the time? So many of my clients get stiff and sore from the workouts I give them, which leads me to remind them to stretch. It seems that although I give my clients homework of taking 10 minutes to stretch after their cardio sessions that I can only get them to do it if I incorporate it into their workouts with me. No, I don't train my clients for cardio. No one needs to pay money to have someone stare at them on a treadmill or elliptical machine.

I've put together a few sequences of very simple yoga stretches that should hit the spot, depending on your needs. These should feel good when you do them. Your body will feel like they need them less and less the more consistent that you are in doing them. In other words, you will feel less stiff over time, but to avoid reversing your progress, you need to continue to do them regardless of if you feel stiff or not. You can't work out whenever you feel out of shape and magically be fit, right? So you can't stretch when you feel stiff and become flexible. Both take time.

You have to find ways to sprinkle in just 10 minutes to keep yourself limber. While you are cooking dinner and your food is simmering. While your kids are playing in the bath. While you are on lunch break at work and you take a stroll to a nearby park. If you make it a habit, you will feel so much better.

All Day At the Office

Spend the morning driving to work, sitting at a desk all day, and then drive home in traffic. Starting to feel like you are taking the shape of a chair? These moves will get your frontside all opened up!

- •. Low Lunge with Lateral Reach: 1 minute each side
- •. Forward Fold with Bind and Twist: 1 minute in fold and 1 minute twisting (2 x each side)
- •. Cat/Cow: 1 minute
- •. Bridge: 1 minute x 2
- •. Reverse Table Top: 1 minute
- •. Supine Twist: 1 minute each side

Cardio Day

Yeah, you're doing cardio! Holy cow, your legs and hips are feeling it. Those big muscles just need some big love. Give them what they crave.

- •. Supine Figure 4: 1 minute each side
- •. Eagle Leg Supine Twist: 1 minute each side
- •. Supine Hamstring Stretch: 1 minute each side
- •. Seated Butterfly: 1 minute
- •. Downward Facing Dog: 1 minute
- •. Supported Camel: 1 minute

Planes, Trains, and Automobiles

Sitting for a long time for business travel or heading somewhere on vacation? Going on a trip can be fun, but it is accompanied with a creaking back and hips that seem to be stuck in place. Move through these poses to feel like less of a tin man and more like Gumby.

- •. Legs Up the Wall: 3 minutes (If your feet are swollen, you may want to put an ice pack wrapped in a towel to further aid in swelling reduction. Once your booty is up against the wall, bend your knees and place the bag on top of your feet, then straighten your legs up the wall.)
- •. Clamshell Twists: 1 and a half minutes per side (30 seconds of movement, 1 minute hold)
- •. Cross-Legged Forward Fold: 1 minute per leg
- •. Reclined Single-Leg Jackknife: 1 minute per leg
- •. Supported Fish: 2 minutes

Yoga exercise references:

Bridge

1. Lie on your back with your knees bent and feet on the floor about hips distance apart.
2. Press through your heels and lift your hips up off of the ground.

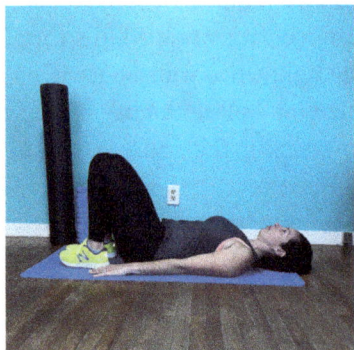

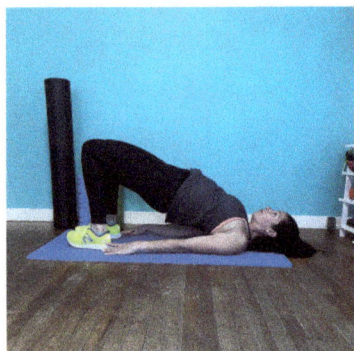

Cat/Cow

1. Get in an all fours position with your shoulders over your wrists and hips over knees.
2. Drop your belly to the ground and lift your tailbone upward while you stretch across your collarbones as if you were trying to pull your chest between your arms.
3. Reverse the position by pulling your belly inward and round your shoulders down towards the ground as you try to exaggerate and arch in your spine.

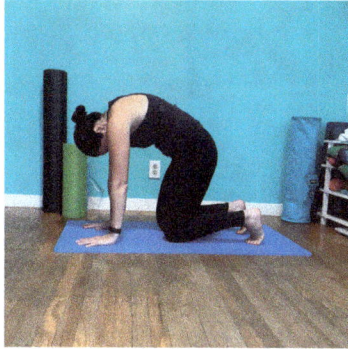

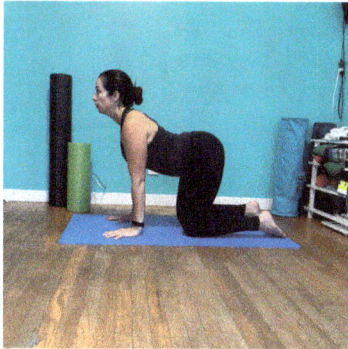

Clamshell Twists

1. Lie on your back with your feet together.
2. Drop both knees over to the right so that the feet and knees are stacked as you are in a gentle twist with the arms in a capital T shape.
3. Bring your left hand to touch your right as you slightly roll to your right side.
4. Open your arms back up to a capital T shape.

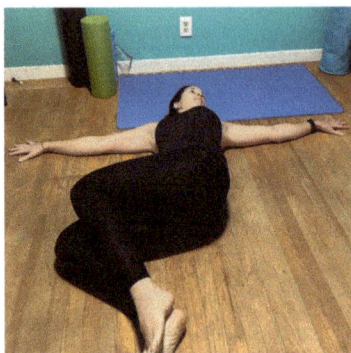

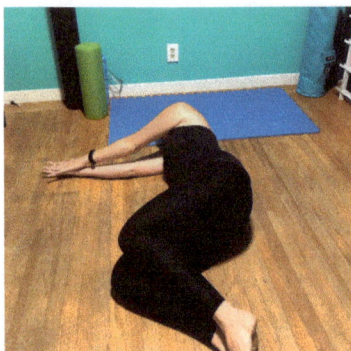

Cross-Legged Forward Fold

1. Stand with your legs hips distance apart.
2. Cross your right leg in front of your left and bend down from the waist.
3. You can use a chair or stool to support you, if needed.
4. Walk your hands to your left to feel more of a stretch in your right hip.
5. Bring your hands back to center and switch sides.

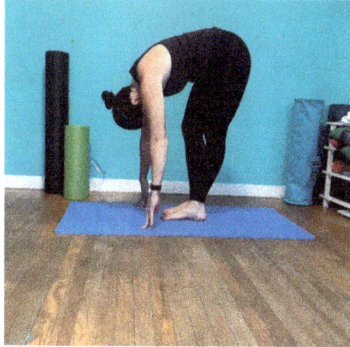

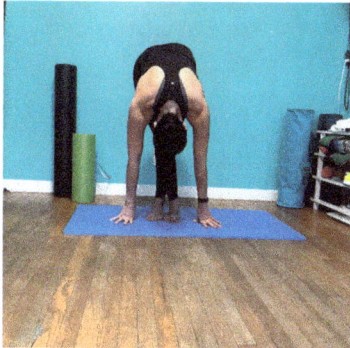

Downward Facing Dog

1. Start in a plank position.
2. Keeping your hands firm on the ground, pull your belly in as you lift your hips up and back.
3. Think about pressing your heels into the ground regardless if they touch to the ground or not.
4. Pull your ribs inwards to prevent arching the lower spine.

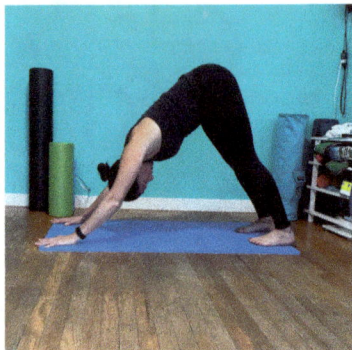

Eagle Leg Supine Twist

1. Lie on your back with your legs in tabletop position so the knees are over the hips with the feet lifted off the ground.
2. With your arms in a capital T position, wrap your right thigh over your left.
3. Drop both knees over to your left side.
4. If the twist feels too deep, you can place a pillow or 2 under your knees.

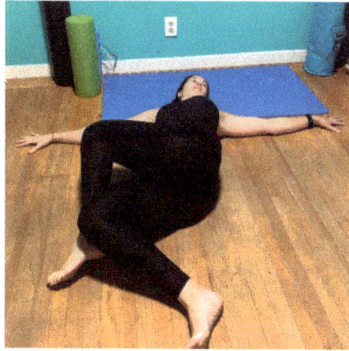

Forward Fold with Bind and Twist

1. Standing with your feet hips distance apart, interlace your fingers behind your back. If you can't interlace your fingers, hold a hand towel or belt in 1 hand and grab it with the other hand behind your back.
2. Fold forward from the waist and let your head drop down.
3. Bend deeply into your left knee as you open your chest over to the right.
4. Switch sides.

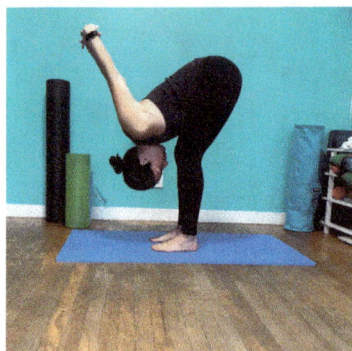

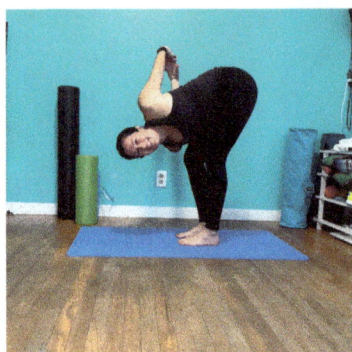

Legs Up the Wall

1. Lie on your back close to a wall.
2. Extend your legs straight up the wall so they can rest.

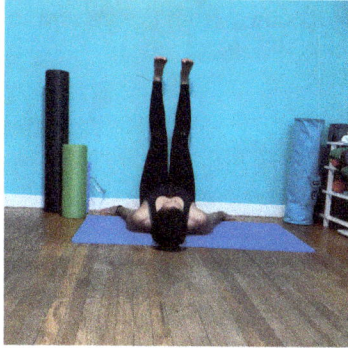

Reverse Table Top

1. Sit on the ground with your feet in front of you at hips distance apart and hands on the ground behind your back with your fingers pointing towards your butt.
2. Lift your hips up slowly from the ground to stretch the front side of your body.

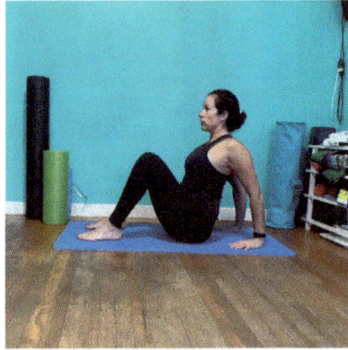

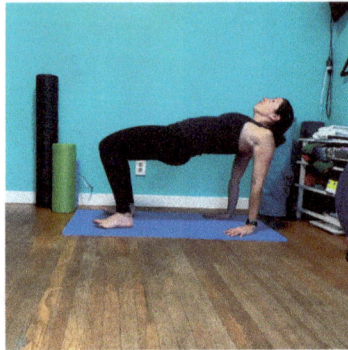

Reclined Single-Leg Jackknife

1. Sitting with both legs extended in front of you, hook your right leg back so that your foot is by your glute.

2. Going slowly, start to lean back any amount to feel the stretch on the top of your right leg.

3. You can also use pillows behind you to help add support and keep you propped up to reduced the intensity of the stretch.

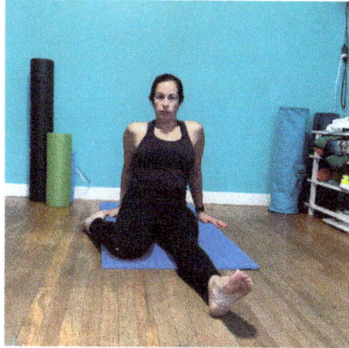

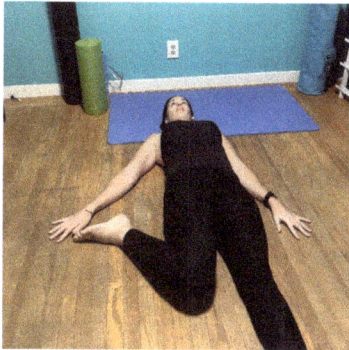

Seated Butterfly

1. From a seated position, bring the soles of your feet together so that your legs are in a butterfly position. The closer your feet are to your groin, the more of a stretch you will get, and the further away, the less of a stretch.
2. Fold over from your waist. For more of a stretch on the inner thigh, keep a flat spine.
3. For more of a stretch in the lower back, round your spine forward.

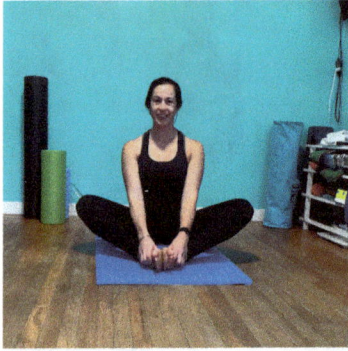

Supine Hamstring Stretch

1. Lie on your back with your knees bent and feet flat on the ground.
2. Extend your leg up in the air and grab behind your leg (if you can't grab your leg, use a towel or belt to wrap behind your leg).
3. Draw your leg towards your chest to stretch the back of your leg.

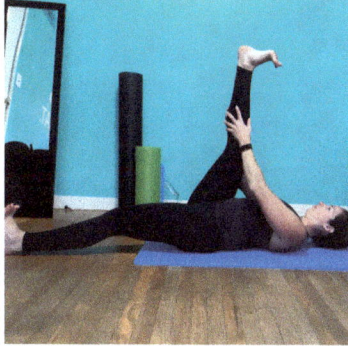

Supine Twist Insert

1. Lie on your back with your arms at a capital T and your knees bent.
2. Lift your feet up off the ground and let your knees drop off to the right, keeping your left shoulder on the ground.
3. Feel free to prop up pillows under your knees if you need less of a twist.

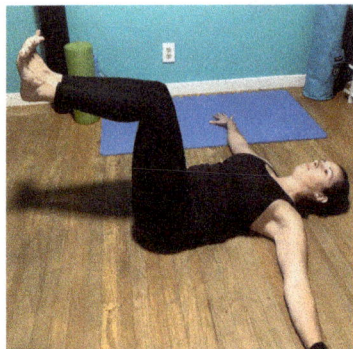

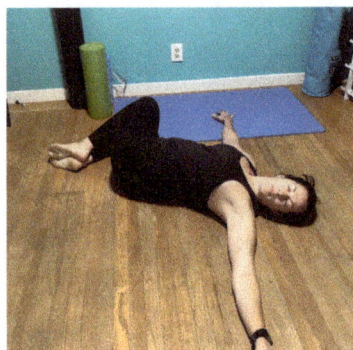

Supine Figure 4

1. Lying on your back with your knees bent and feet flat on the floor, cross your right ankle on top of your left thigh.
2. Reach your right hand between your legs and left hand to the outer left thigh to pull your left leg in towards your chest.
3. You will feel the stretch on the outer right hip.

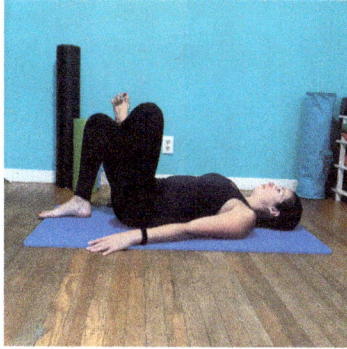

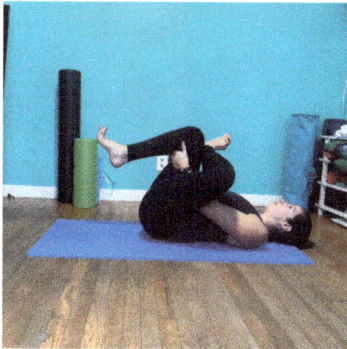

Supported Camel

1. From a kneeling position, place your hands to your lower back.
2. Start to lean back some to feel a stretch across the entire front of your body.
3. Think about keeping any bend to the mid-back as to protect the lower back.
4. Very slowly, roll back up and sit back on your heels.

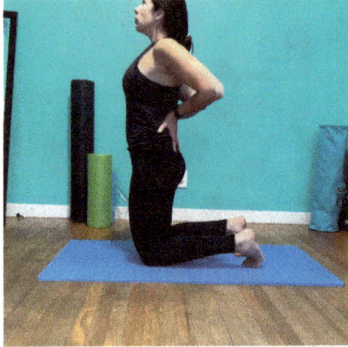

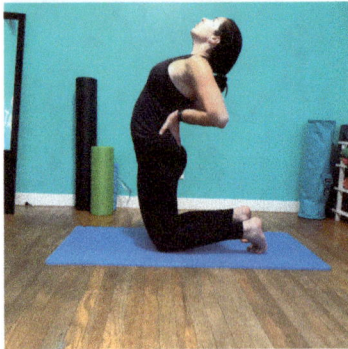

Supported Fish

1. Sit down on the ground with your legs extended in front of you.
2. Place your fingers under your butt and slowly lean back so that you are supported on your forearms.
3. You can drop the crown of your head back onto the ground or a pillow.

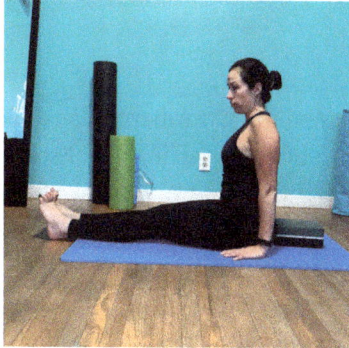

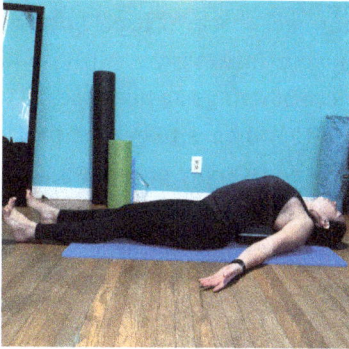

$\mathcal{SMR}$

No, SMR doesn't stand for "Strawberry Mango Frosting" (although that sounds really good!). I'm talking about self-myofascial release. Who can say that 5 times fast? We'll stick with SMR for now. The reason I want you to know about SMR and why it is so important is because stretching alone is not enough to take care of the muscles in your body. MANY people think that it is enough.

Let me ask you this, have you ever had a knot in a muscle before? Maybe around your neck, back, or legs? I don't know you, but I'm going to guess that your answer is yes. Most people have. Now if you have a knot in a piece of string or a necklace, do you pull on it to get it out? Of course not! You have to get the tangle out. To untangle your muscles, you need to apply pressure and massage techniques in and around that adhesion to get it to relax and eventually release. Ultimately, you can remove the adhesion and gain full function of your muscle again.

Beginning a new healthy lifestyle will mean that you will start to use muscles that you never even knew you had. They are going to get cranky after a while the more you use them. You could get a massage a couple of times a week, but if you are reading this book because you are trying to be healthier with little time or money, then making multiple trips to the spa every week isn't going to work. There are several tools out there on the market, but I will share with you my ultimate go-to. Yoga Tune Up therapy balls. I use these not only for myself, but I have used them with each and every one of my clients in some capacity. They are inexpensive, portable, and easy-to-use. To explore different areas of your body and a multitude of ways to use them, I would recommend getting "The Roll Model" by Jill Miller. This woman is completely brilliant in teaching people how to use these balls to feel better with their bodies (she is also the creator of these miracle balls). Although I have not had the pleasure of studying directly under her, I have studied with others that are students of hers. There are many tools out there like foam rollers to use, but I truly enjoy using these specific tools to address my body's needs.

When you are first starting out with SMR, I would say to just explore all over your body. You can take about 5 to 7 deep breaths for each muscle before moving on to the next. If you have the time, you can explore every muscle in your body. Start by applying pressure to the muscle by either lying over the ball facedown or face up. Take a few deep breaths here. Roll the balls over the muscle and experiment moving them in a variety of directions. If you don't massage your entire body at one time, just do a different part every day for around 10 minutes. You can pair this with your physical activity or a way to relax before bed.

Most muscles can be accessed by rolling around on the floor, but if you find this too intense, feel free to take the balls to the wall to alleviate the amount of pressure you are applying. Make sure that you continue to breathe as you massage. If the muscle is so tight that you are holding your breath, you may want to back off and massage around that spot instead.

There are a few places that you want to avoid placing the balls. Most of these will seem like common sense and had me laughing during training thinking, "Who the heck would put the ball there?" I just want to make sure that you stay safe and avoid injuring yourself over something like self-massage.

Places to avoid placing the Yoga Tune Up Balls:

- •. Throat
- •. Breastbone
- •. Underside of wrist in extension: Achieved by laying your palm face down and then pointing your fingers upward.
- •. Hamstrings with straight leg: This will feel painful as you hit your sciatic nerve. Massage hamstrings always with a bent knee on a chair or kneeling.
- •. Tailbone: You can laugh and shake your head! I did!
- •. An active injury
- •. Bruised tissue, broken bones, or open wounds
- •. Any area that causes a feeling of sharp pain

Deep pressure to these areas could cause pain, discomfort, and/or injury.

Reinventing Your Wheel

As you start to incorporate these new habits into your life, you will encounter bumps along the way. This not only happens now but throughout your life. As I wrote this book, I also struggled to find time to train my clients, eat, shower, sleep, and work out. The daily activities are so basic, yet if you throw in a curveball, everything all of a sudden seems impossible. When this happens, you need to do what you did when you first opened this book. Look at your situation, find the time that you do have free, and work with what you have.

There may be times when you only have 20 or 30 minutes in your day to work out. So then just do 30 minutes. Make the best use of your time by taking shorter breaks between your exercises. If you are doing cardio, just throw in a few higher intensity bursts. Life isn't perfect, but finding opportunities to sprinkle in your fitness when you can will keep you with the right mindset. It will always be at the forefront of your mind to do something healthy for yourself versus it being just an afterthought.

When the going gets tough, take these steps to re-evaluate and get your wheel spinning again:

Review your goals: Sometimes we aren't able to find time because we have met our goals or they need to be revisited. Maybe the goals you set were too broad or too long term. Set smaller goals to help you regain focus and make it feel easy to step back in the right direction.

Reset your workout days: If your work schedule has changed or it's summer and the kids now have soccer practice, then you may find that your free time has shifted. There may be other things that need to move to accommodate your time to get your sweat on, but just do it. You won't regret it.

Lean on your support system: Ask for support from your friends, family, spouse, or co-workers. This can come in many different forms depending on the help you need. It is likely that someone close to you will also be needing support, so return the favor. Maybe you have a friend that needs someone to watch her kids so she can get in a jog. You can trade off or get together with your kids and do a fun family-friendly workout together. Don't be afraid to ask for help. It doesn't make you weak; it's representative of the amazing circle of support that you are surrounded by.

Swirl and Shake

The longer you go developing a regular routine of working out and trying new things, being physically active may start to feel like a chore. Something new always feels exciting, right? You can think of your new healthy lifestyle like you would a new relationship. When you start a new relationship, you aren't quite sure where things are going to lead, but you are having fun getting to try new stuff out and exploring areas of yourself that you weren't aware that you liked. You feel like you are on cloud nine and a whole new you is born.

Then the honeymoon phase is over. Things are slightly uncomfortable at times. You aren't sure if you really like this new thing anymore, and you may even miss your old life a bit. Just like a relation-ship when the going gets tough, and you want to throw in the towel, you will feel the same way about your relationship with healthy food, exercises, and the new lifestyle in general. Sometimes an old routine feels so comfortable that it is just easier to have that old way of life back. The thing is that you decided to make positive changes in your way of living because it was no longer serving you. Go back to your why from the start of this book.

Just like the relationship that starts to go stale, you will want to shake things up a bit. I am constantly looking for new inspiration to keep things from getting boring. My job requires me to train clients all day. If I don't keep things a bit interesting, I would have zero mo-tivation to do anything for myself.

My top 5 ways to shake things up:
1. **Change your environment**. If you work out in a gym, try taking your sessions outdoors. If you workout solo, then take a group fitness class. Having different scenery can make things have a fresh new feeling even if you are doing almost the same thing.
2. **New fitness equipment**. Some fitness equipment is ridicu-lous in price. I swear, the price tag goes up 10-fold because it is for fitness. Try using paper plates on carpet or socks on hardwood floor for fitness gliders. Grab your kids skateboard to do ab rollouts or put one foot on for single-leg squats. There are a ton of household items that you can use to make your workout more interesting. Get creative!
3. **Try a new recipe**. Has there been a food you have been curi-ous about? Bok choy, Swiss chard, pomegranate, or persim-mon? Look up a recipe, and make something new! The fun about exploring is finding new things that you like. How will you know if you stick to the same old things? Be adventurous and open to new flavors that may just tickle your taste buds.
4. **Join a group**. You can explore a variety of ways to be physi-cally fit through various social groups. Many companies have groups that get together to play softball, flag football, or that

provide group exercise like yoga. Companies today are more and more inclined to provide ways to keep their employees healthy. You may also find something of interest online with a forum like MeetUp.com. Many of these groups are affordable, such as my donation-based yoga class that I offer here in Mountain View, California. If you are in the area look, me up on MeetUp.com under "Get Fit In The Park."

5. **Bump that beat.** Finding some of your favorite songs to work out to can help make the time go by like the speed of lightning. I also like listening to music when I am in the kitchen cooking. Music just speaks to my soul, and I tend to enjoy things more when I am having fun with good music coming out of the speakers. Find what moves you on the inside and use it to add some enjoyment into everything that you do.

Conclusion: The
Whole Enchilada

Look at you! How cool is it that you have come this far. You have made so many changes in your life and are turning into this amazingly strong and health-oriented new person. I am seriously so proud of you for taking this huge first step. Be proud of yourself too. So many people would give up on themselves, but you didn't.

Knowing Your Why

Remember why you want to be healthy, fit, and strong. What is important to me may not be the same things that are important to you. Reflect on your Board of Reason to give you strength to do workouts when you would rather skip and rest. Being healthy means that you are just finding ways to sprinkle in fitness and nutrition throughout the day. If you attempt to be perfect you won't be. Don't put that pressure on yourself cause it's not important to find perfection. Focus on making tiny changes every day and eventually you will have evolved into someone that puts their well-being first while still having fun.

Cleaning From the Inside Out

You know that feeling good starts with what you put into your body. Surround yourself with nutrient dense foods and keep the crappy stuff out of your house. Ask for the support of your family and friends to not pressure you back into poor eating habits. Explain to them your why and how come you want to be a healthier version of yourself. Whether it is because you want to be a better parent, return to the athlete you once were, or prevent hereditary disease, those that surround you will not only embrace you with support but may feel inspired to want to lead a healthier life like you have chosen for yourself.

Eating better has a lot to do with planning. Take foods you like and add more nutrients to them like veggies or healthy fats. Remove items with processed sugar and stuff that can last years on a shelf. Fresh food is not only better for you but tastes delicious on your lips. Share these new recipe twists with your family and friends. Growing up, I was rarely exposed to these types of nutritious foods. You have the opportunity right here right now to break the cycle and influence those around you to potentially live well in their bodies.

Move Freely

Finding new ways to move your body can be a fun and exploratory process. Learning how to challenge yourself safely in ways that you never have before can at times feel frustrating and almost impossible, but the very word impossible spells I-AM-POSSIBLE. Somedays you won't have a ton of time to dedicate to a full workout. If you do 15 minutes, then that's what you get in. Life will get in the way, however, putting yourself first on your schedule will keep you feeling worthy and energized.

Utilize the exercises in this book and know that you can do them anywhere simply with just your bodyweight. Getting fit doesn't require you to pay for a gym membership or the latest equipment. When looking to intensify your workouts, think about using things around your house such as canned goods, milk jugs, or even your kids for extra weight. Lock down the fundamental movements with good form before making things more challenging. This will ensure your success as you get stronger and discover your inner athlete.

Filling In the Gap

Proper nutrition and exercise can be the obvious focal points when it comes to creating a healthier lifestyle. Don't forget that there are other aspects that will help to support your new nutrition and exercise choices. Remembering to drink enough water in order to replenish lost fluids from working out will be an important addition along with getting enough sleep. Both of these will help to regulate your hunger hormones so you eat to provide fuel for your body and not out of boredom or in an effort to stay awake.

Other methods of self-care such as massage, yoga, and meditation will balance out the influx of energy by creating a sense of calm. Your body needs to be taken care of in a gentle way just as much as it needs a little push in those workouts. Giving yourself some TLC will generate that sense of balance your body craves to continue to do this for many years to come.

Let's Take a Look At How Far You've Come

Write down 3 new habits that you have developed that have a positive impact on your health:

1. _____

2. _____

3. _____

What is 1 improvement you have noticed within yourself since you have started this program?

_____

Name 1 thing that you feel you could continue to improve upon?

_____

Now look in the mirror and tell yourself:

*"You are capable
and worthy of living a fun2befit life!"*

Fitness Inspiration

Corporate Success

Romi Simpson is a 40-year-old chief of staff for a moderately sized bank. Having spent her college years and beyond in London, Romi was very use to walking as a means of transportation. After relocating to the United States, she found herself initially with a commute to and from work while she was pinned to a desk all day. Eventually, she knew things were going to have to change by finding a way to add more movement back into her day.

Upon receiving a promotion, Romi decided to find a place to live that was walking distance to work as well as places to enjoy in her free time. With a 30-minute walk to and from work, she is able to log 12 to 15 thousand steps per day according to her Fitbit. This walk also serves as meditation time, she can walk into the office with a sense of calm and let any work related stress be resolved on her way home.

Banking On Your Health

Prior to starting a personal training program, Ida Valentine, a 23-year-old investment banker, rarely ate her greens. Vegetables were a mere afterthought as her main focus during meal time was protein, carbs, and of course dessert. The thing was, Ida didn't have a good idea as to what a healthy meal looked like. She knew that vegetables were good for her, but how much should she eat?

Through constant interaction with her trainer, Christine Oakes, she realized that aiming for half of what she consumes should be vegetables and fruits. Ida was able to have a clearer picture on how to construct a nutritious meal by shifting the ratios of her meals. Today, Ida may not be perfect, however, making these adjustments has made a noticeable difference in how she feels every day.

Endorphin Bliss

Sometimes personal failures can put us in a state of despair that we forget how to take care of ourselves. After going through a break-up, Maxim Ossipov, a 32-year-old software engineer, realized that he needed to try something new. He decided to go to a yoga class while he was living in New York City. $40 bought him an entire month of yoga.

Maxim felt slightly out of place as he was surrounded by younger, more fit yogis that all seemed to know what they were doing. He tried to just follow along and by the end of the class he was hooked. After his first yoga experience, Maxim remembers clearly how calm his mind felt as he was intoxicated with endorphins, bliss, and focus. By being present in the moment, he was able to let his brain stop feeling so overwhelmed and realized what was important. Putting yourself first!

Christine's Wellness Must-Haves

These are just some of my favorite things that I enjoy using on a regular basis. I thought I would put together a little list for you so you can explore what you like and eventually have your own list of must-haves.

Food:

Amy's veggie burgers, burritos, and soups: www.amys.com
Arbonne protein powder: www.christineoakes.arbonne.com
Costco salmon, canned beans, salsa, avocado oil, frozen fruits and veggies: www.costco.com
Ezekial bread: www.foodforlife.com
Gardein meatless products: www.gardein.com
Hinode microwaveable rice: www.hinoderice.com
Kind bars (almond and coconut is my favorite!!): www.kindbars.com
Miyoko's vegan cheese: www.miyokoskitchen.com

Sabra hummus cups: www.sabra.com
Trader Joe's: almond butter, falafel, hummus (so many yummy flavors including edamame), olive oil, low-sodium pasta sauce, quinoa duo with vegetable melange, trail mix

Note: Many of these foods can be found in your local grocer. Since there are many grocery stores across the country and world, I thought it would be more useful to give you links for the products so you know what you are looking for when you go shopping. Some vendors do sell their products online as well as Amazon (www.amazon.com) tends to also sell many things found in stores.

Gadgets
Body fat scale by 1byOne: www.amazon.com
Nutribullet: www.nutribullet.com

Apps
Accountability by Dietbet and Gym-pact
Meditation by Calm and Headspace

Accessories
Freezeable lunch box by Packit: www.packit.com
Yoga mats: www.gaiam.com
Yoga Tune Up balls: www.yogatuneup.com

Clothes
Old Navy: www.oldnavy.com
Target: www.target.com

Books

Journey to the Heart by Melody Beatie
The 4-Hour Workweek by Tim Ferris
The Roll Model by Jill Miller

Find all books on www.amazon.com

Other

Kis Essential Oils: www.kisoils.com
Onlywax soy candle: www.amazon.com
Spotify music: www.spotify.com